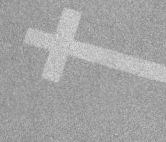

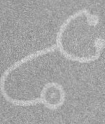

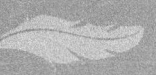

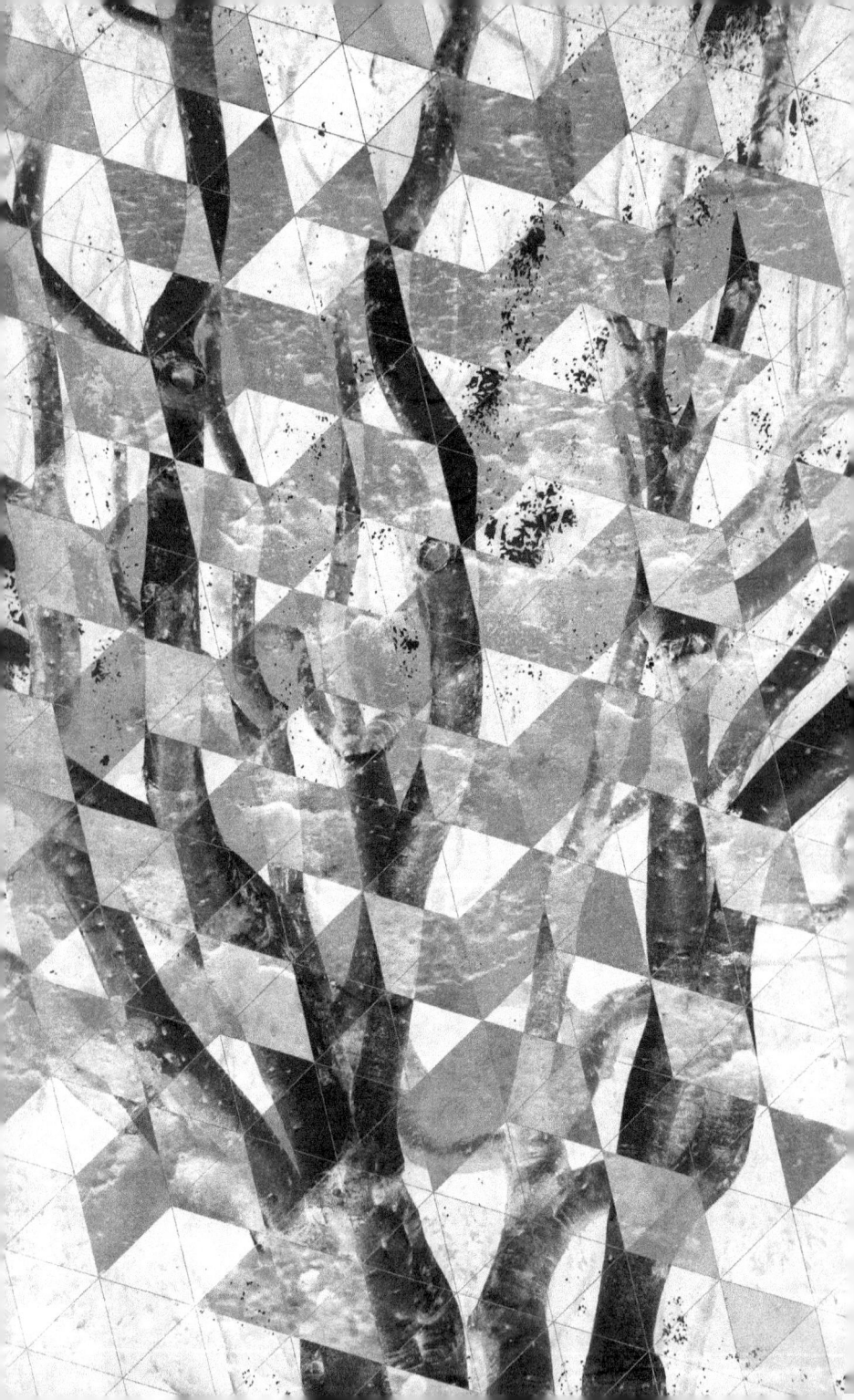

The Evolve Fertility Series
by Beth Alderman, MD, MPH

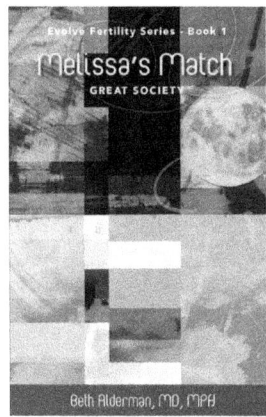

Evolve Fertility Series - Book 1
Melissa's Match
GREAT SOCIETY

Beth Alderman, MD, MPH

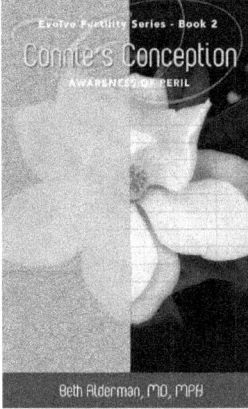

Evolve Fertility Series - Book 2
Corinne's Conception
AWARENESS OF PERIL

Beth Alderman, MD, MPH

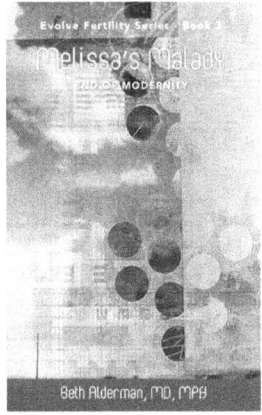

Evolve Fertility Series - Book 3
Melissa's Malady
END OF MODERNITY

Beth Alderman, MD, MPH

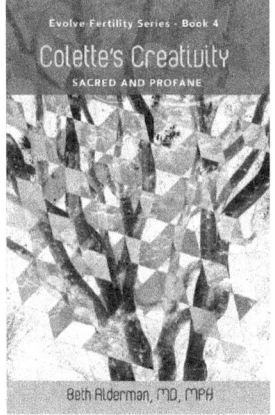

Evolve Fertility Series - Book 4
Colette's Creativity
SACRED AND PROFANE

Beth Alderman, MD, MPH

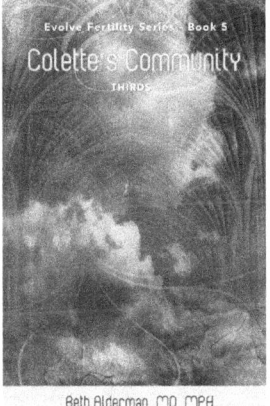

Evolve Fertility Series - Book 5
Colette's Community
THIRDS

Beth Alderman, MD, MPH

Colette's Creativity

SACRED AND PROFANE

Book Four of the
Evolve Fertility Series

Beth Alderman, MD, MPH

LIVING FUTURE BOOKS • ASHLAND, OREGON

Colette's Creativity: Sacred and Profane
by Beth Alderman, MD, MPH
© 2019 Future Medicine, LLC
www.LivingFutureBooks.com

For related online courses visit
www.LivingFutureCourses.com

Editor: Julie Clayton
Cover Art: www.BruceBayard.com
Book Design: www.BookSavvyStudio.com

Library of Congress Control Number: 2019903851
ISBN: 978-1-7321110-3-5
First Edition
Printed in the United States of America

Contents

To Nancy and Stephanie

It's only castles burning,
Find someone who's turning,
And we will come around.
                    —NEIL YOUNG

1

Runaway

On Monday morning, when Andy and I return to St. Kilda from the Prahran market where we bought supplies, Reggie says, "Your friend Melissa called from the States. You're to call right away. Use Mum's phone; Andy and I'll run down the checklist, make sure we have what we need."

I do not feel ready to talk to Melissa, my childhood friend. At the same time, I am secretly pleased that she went to so much trouble to find me overseas, in Australia. I go into Reggie's mum's bedroom, close the door, and find the phone. I smooth my long raven hair and eyebrows and check my violet eyes, pale skin, and shiny teeth in the mirror so that I will feel put together when we speak. Then I dial.

"Colette! Are you all right? We've all been worried sick!"

Hearing my friend's anxiety, I visualize her eyes accusing me, and I feel helpless. I take a deep breath and promise myself to take it slow, to avoid the old habit of surrendering to her will.

"How did you find me?"

"Steve called last week. He said you'd disappeared. We all thought you'd been kidnapped. We couldn't imagine how or where you could have gone. And then I remembered your friend Reggie the winemaker, and started calling around to wine stores down there in Melbourne, and finally found a clerk who recognized her name, and who told me she was at Denton Stables. I looked it up on the web, and called their number, and they gave me this number. And now here you are sounding fine! What were you thinking? How could you just abandon all your responsibilities?"

The other side of the world is suddenly far too near. I sit for a moment, speechless, stuck between past and present. Then I say, "It's good to hear your voice. Thank you for taking the trouble to find me."

Melissa continues, "I can't tell you what a relief it is to hear *your* voice! Are you okay?" After a brief pause in which I try to picture her point of view and to organize a response, she declares, "Talk to me, Colette! What's going on?"

"I'm fine. I'm going to help Reggie's family set up a new business."

"Fine? You can't be! You left your husband for her! Are you in love with her?"

"What? No!"

"Is this a midlife crisis? Are you trying to punish Steve?"

"I've left Steve. I plan to work here until I figure out what's next."

"Steve called and asked me if you had run off to join some kind of a lesbian cult. He must have called your mom, because when I called her, she was so hysterical she couldn't speak English! I had to call your brother, and he said your mom lit enough candles to fill Notre Dame. He had no idea what was going on—though he did say you were unhappy with Steve, which is something you never told me."

Her accusations burn. I try to put myself in her place, but I can't. I brace myself to set limits on her reaction. "I wish you would give me the benefit of the doubt! I never wanted or expected to live with his bitter family. I was dying inside. I told you what it was like and you never wanted to hear it. Reggie was the only one who listened and accepted and understood."

Melissa's voice shifts. "I didn't want to be the kind of friend who would stand by and watch you throw away twenty years of marriage."

"I didn't want you to be the kind of friend who would stand by and watch me wither in a dead marriage until it was too late to start over."

There is a long silence.

I continue, "I could really use your support now. See if you can respect my feelings and my decisions. Assume I know what I'm doing and am solving my problems, until you find out otherwise."

"Colette, every week for twenty years you told me the good and funny things in your life. Now you act like they never happened. I feel like I don't know who you are."

My will and Melissa's are colliding in a painful way; our old connection has let us down. To mend it, I must establish a better one. "Many marriages break down. Mine did. Friends face the hard times as well as the good ones."

"What should I do?"

"Start by sitting down and writing me a nice long email about what's happening in your life, and then I'll reply by telling you what's happening in mine, and we'll take it from there. And please accept that this is a difficult time for me and that I could use your support."

"Alright. But how will I—how will I know what you're leaving out?"

"Hopefully I won't leave things out, and you won't filter them out."

"What about your mom, and Steve?"

"Let me worry about them. And please don't give them this number."

"All right. All right. If that's what you want. But be careful, okay? It's dangerous down there with all those snakes and sharks and spiders. Do you know the injury rates to surfers down there?"

Her concern touches me. It is poignant, and amusing. I smile. "Thanks for taking time to track me down. I don't want to burn this bridge. I just need to make some changes, deep ones, and I don't have a map or a story to guide me. I'm taking it one step at a time."

Melissa pledges her support. We exchange long and reluctant Midwestern farewells, taking care to assuage hurt feelings and to affirm mutual affection. We are like Japanese elders who take turns bowing lower and lower to be sure they have shown each other sufficient respect. And then we hang up and I am left standing in my new life, unsteady from the encroachment of the old one.

I stand and look into a mirror that hangs between the bed and the window, put the phone to my ear, and practice what I want to say to Steve.

"I spent two decades doing something I never wanted to do, and decided not to continue."

Too distant, too sterile, too selfish. The story of our life together belongs to both of us.

"I wish you hadn't given up on our plans so early on."

Too whiny.

"You and your mother threw away our plans for starting a

4

business with the excuse that you were rescuing a dying family farm that neither of you had the guts to change."

Too self-righteous.

"I'm sorry. I just couldn't stay."

Too defeatist.

I accept that I will have to wing it. To tell Steve a story, I would have to grasp what happened between us, and I don't. Not yet. I pick up the receiver and brace myself to dial. Before I'm remotely ready, I find myself saying, "Hello, Steven."

After an unpleasant pause, he rasps, "What happened to you?"

I am not prepared for the timbre of his voice, nor for the wave of nostalgia it raises. I feel as if I am right back on our sofa, sitting next to him in the evening, nudging him awake after he's fallen asleep. In the background, the television is assaulting us with programming I detest. The comfort of the familiar meets the dull knife of pent-up misery. I feel a pang of regret and a spin of confusion. I hear myself ask tenderly, "Are you all right?"

"You left Mom's truck at the airport! We didn't get any work done at all that day."

This anger and blame are nothing special; what is new is that I no longer accept them. I did everything I could and he stonewalled me. The solution of creative expression was mine. It could have been ours, had he been willing. But he wasn't. He continued to obey his parents' will, and to deny the all-pervasive forces driving family farms like theirs into oblivion. The more he failed, the more he took it out on me. In the present, I take a deep breath and notice that his only concern now, as always, is himself.

"I'm not asking for a settlement, Steve."

"Are you—does that woman have you sleeping with her?"

"That woman has me working for her. It's a summer job."

"What the hell are you doing, Colette! You *have* a job! For Christ's sake, Mom's been cleaning and cooking, and Dad and I are swamped. How could you think we'd cope while you went gallivanting away? Where are you, anyway?"

I feel the pull of duty and the long habit of looking after farm and family. I realize that I am still staring at my reflection and that I can't tell whether I'm laughing or crying. I was their work horse as well as their scapegoat. I did not run from Steven; I ran from my old self. I am mute.

Steven continues. "It's time you came back and faced up to your responsibilities."

"I can't do it anymore, Steve. I wanted to leave for years, and I finally got up the gumption. I'm not coming back. I want a divorce."

"Oh, that old stuff. You're always nagging—" he stops short. I can tell that he is working hard to mind his words. "Well, if I'd known you were fed up we could have taken a little trip when things slowed down."

"Things never *do* slow down. Which is odd, because they're always slow."

"Do you know how selfish you are? You want this and you want that. You're not the only one that doesn't get what you want!"

"By your account, what I want is selfish and what you want is necessary. I'm sorry I put up with that."

"You're selfish and you know it!"

I laugh. I would never have done that at home; I would have been too afraid. But now, for the first time, I feel safe from neglect and spite. "Steve, I hear nothing in what you've said to suggest that you value what you lost, by which I mean me, or that you might have done anything to cause me to leave, or that you might be willing to change. All I hear is the usual whining abuse. What woman in her right mind would return to that?"

"When I think of how I could have had Candace I—I—"

"Candace?" I picture Candace in her faux Nashville clothes and teased black hair. I see her pouty mouth pouring out petty, divisive intrigues. I see destruction in her wake. I see Steven seeing none of it. "What do you mean could have had her?"

"She wanted to run off, but I said no, we had to stick it out. I'm not like you. I live up to my responsibilities!"

I remember that shortly after Candace affected a southern twang, Steven did too. "You plugged Candace?"

"You don't know how many offers I've had! Men my age have their pick. Women your age are desperate. You'll have your way, all right. You'll live alone and die alone."

I almost step on the merry-go-round. I open my mouth to say, "By the way, Steve, it's your mother's fault," but I catch myself before any sound comes out. I can think of many wrong things to say, but no right ones. I rummage my brain for a storyline and find only the old existential version of our lives in which Steven and I loved each other but drifted apart due to deep, mysterious differences in our souls. I know that the truth is grittier and nastier than that. It would be more accurate to say that we bumbled blindly along, spoiling each other's happiness until the lights of our hearts nearly went out. And then it dawns on me. Steve gave me the perfect reason. I am tempted to hang up right now and call Melissa back to tell her that Stephen was unfaithful.

"Oh, Steve, thank God! Thank you for telling me."

"What? What's that supposed to mean? Did you— Did you—?"

"No! I've been feeling guilty, and ashamed, and now I don't have to. You broke the marriage contract! Some part of me must have known that."

"What do you mean? It was your fault! You never gave me what I needed!"

I smile. I can't help it. I feel giddy. "Can't you see? I've done us both a favor. I set you free! My hopes and dreams will no longer trouble you. They're mine, and mine alone. Plus you chose it first, which will make it easier to be friends."

"Friends? Why should we be friends? We don't even like each other. We just—we're family, not friends."

"I filed for divorce. The papers are on their way. If you sign them, you'll make this easier on both of us. I hope you find someone soon."

I ring off. I disconnect to save him from hearing the retorts that encircle my mind like a flaming crown of thorns. *He's such an asshole! Asshole, asshole, asshole!* My thoughts go on a rant about Everything That's Wrong With Steven, about how he is a momma's boy who's never grown up, and who never will.

And then I see it. If he is a black hole of unhappiness, I am one of disappointment. For fifteen years, I have been unable to see him as a lover, potential father, or companion. I failed to free him from his greatest fear, the fear that poverty may cost him his patrimony, that a thoughtlessly constructed strip mall would obliterate the land cultivated by his forebears. How could I free him? But in failing to free him, I failed to free myself. I felt manipulated, oppressed, and put upon. I believed I was powerless and had no choice but to accept my fate. And then, suddenly and without warning, I abandoned him to defeat. How terrible for him.

"No, I am the asshole!" I whisper. I hear Maman's voice telling me that marriage is once and only once, and that it is up to the wife to make it work. I feel a stab of guilt and an impulse to treat this like a vacation. I could return to Steve and try again. *No, no! This is the problem. I mustn't take responsibility for his errors as well as mine. I mustn't treat him like a child.* I have to finally say no to him in a way that cannot be misconstrued by either of us.

And I have to tell my mother that I am doing it. That will be the hardest part. None of my years of centering prayer, nor the building of equanimity, nor practicing love of the enemy, nor leading Quaker-sponsored peacebuilding efforts in areas of conflict—none of these has prepared me to cope with my mother. Her influence over me—her presence in me—is too strong. Maman is devoted to what she sees as the One True Church; she obeys the letter of its laws. She may never accept the dissolution of my marriage. I dial her number slowly, hoping that Andy or Reggie will interrupt me.

"Allo?"

I can see Maman sitting on the brown sofa in the living room of our brick ranch-style home in Peoria. She'll have spread a quilt over the worn, shiny spot on the cushion nearest the telephone, where she sits when she's gossiping with friends from church. I sit on my bed as if I am in the easy chair opposite her and continue in Acadian French. "Maman? Melissa called. She said that you might be worried."

"Colette! Mon Dieu! Tell me that you've come to your senses, and that you will be returning to your husband!"

Her dramatic tone sweeps away time and distance. I am back in the kitchen looking up at Maman as she justifies scolding me by invoking an inscrutable Catholic doctrine. Any effort

I make to explain or to protest will invite further scolding for disobedience. I want to leave the kitchen, but I am too obedient. I had to become desperate before I could work up the courage to defy her. In my teen years, I accepted the role of sinner and found the courage to talk back. Later, I taught myself to accept and love her as she is, to be grateful for her dignity and duty. And yet now I find myself losing my poise: I fall back into the role of guilty scapegoat and respond in the sardonic tone of my teens.

"Maman, I'm not here by accident! I came of my own free will."

Maman does not reply.

"I suppose you'd rather I'd been kidnapped?"

"How could you endanger your immortal soul?"

I stand and look at the mirror for moral support. "Listen, I know you want me to go to hell, but do you mind if I wait a few years?"

"My only daughter has fallen willingly into mortal sin! I'm so ashamed."

"You can't be surprised! Sin was the number one topic at the dinner table."

"You even mock God!"

"No, Maman," I say, failing to keep my voice calm. "I mock the idea that there can be only one opinion on the subject of divorce. And I refuse to accept that the woman should stay no matter what."

"You shouldn't have married outside the faith! That's how you learned these terrible things."

"Maman, all my life I've been obedient to the point of being irresponsible. I need to take charge of my life. I shouldn't have run away, but I knew how you'd take my decision, and I didn't know what else to do."

"You can't find your way if you're angry with God."

Maman said the same thing when I complained about parochial school, when I left the Church, and again when I married into a family of anti-papist Congregationalists.

"I wish I could make this easier for you."

"You shouldn't put this terrible burden on me. I'm too old."

"I'm sorry, Maman, but I'm finally doing the right thing and I don't think that should be a burden to you. And I'll try not to take it personally that you want me to go to hell. Okay, listen, I'll call you again when I'm feeling stronger."

"There's no telling whether I'll be around. You'll be the death of me."

I sigh and slump. My maturity failed, but I can at least avoid the old game of vying for biggest victim. "Take care of yourself, my dear Maman. And don't worry about me, okay? I'll be fine."

"What can I say?"

"You can tell me that you love me and wish me the best."

Maman is silent. I asked for this curse of omission, but it hurts all the same. "I love you, Ma. A bientôt."

I hang up. I feel the role of child pulling at me. It is my former self, hoping to please Maman, who has not changed her tactics since she pulled my hair during Mass to keep me still. She hasn't had to change her tactics; they still work. *It's because I'm not a mother. It's because I have no child.*

That's what Maman wants for me, deep down, and I sometimes think that's what I want, too. Mostly I see that as a weakness in both my mother and myself. I pull myself up and remember to be determined to take my perilous turn at finding my path. Once I have, I will do my part to give birth to the mysterious and unforeseeable future.

2

Single

For the next few days, as jet lag drags me down, I follow Reggie on her rounds of urban family and business connections while Andy disappears into his home neighborhood of North Melbourne. Each new Aussie face I encounter expresses a fresh concoction of the local ways of sharing thoughts and showing feelings. At first, the nuances escape me, but soon I begin to absorb the manners and mores, and to build the mid-Pacific persona that brings me closer to creating a new and better life—a new and better me.

On the weekend, we make the rounds of Reggie's oldest friends, beginning with an early dinner at her favorite pub with her mates from the University of Melbourne, which she calls Uni. During the week, I'd felt like an iron woman dashing across St. Kilda's beach, lurching through deep sand and sloshing in shallow water. Now I plunge into the raucous sea of nightlife in which I am a curiosity, watching the scene and sipping a pint as I get my bearings and feel my way into a social niche that will allow me a place in the group.

"The Espy's a historic place," says Roger. He waves an arm expansively, nearly knocking over his wife Judy's glass. "The Gold Rush started here. A bloke came back from California and told the crowd at the bar that we had the same kind of rock as they did, and probably had gold ore, too. They laughed him out of the pub. So up he went to Ballarat, and the bastard struck gold and made it rich."

"The Espy was built thirty years after that," Judy says mildly.

"And the literati frequent the place now," continues Roger blithely, taking a drag of his cigarette and blowing its smoke over his plate of pub food. "Robert Hughes always staggers across Albert Square, pissing on that statue or the palm tree. The bugger's never sober."

"You saw him once, Rog," Judy observes, putting an ashtray under Roger's cigarette.

"You're spoiling my stories, doll, nothing wrong with a good story. Sells real estate. Keeps you in sherry, doesn't it?"

"Botrytis," I pipe up. "Reggie wants us all to drink her Botrytis."

"Hal woult say that story iss all that matterss," says Dutchy in her thick accent. "History ass we know it is just a construct that winners create to seem virtuouss, or inevitable."

"Hal is a sociology professor and a postmodernist," Judy explains smoothly. "And we all admire his ground-breaking work."

"I see. Well, we didn't have a lot of constructs back in Maine. A dead chicken is pretty much a dead chicken, and a bad year is a bad year," I say.

Roger laughs. "And a pint of Cooper's is a good one, and not a construct of one."

"So tell me about your construct of an Australian," I say to Judy. "I've been trying to figure out how Australians differ from Americans. At first I thought it was the freckles, but now I'm thinking it's the alcohol. I've never seen so many drink so much, and I'm Irish!"

"I'll tell you," Roger replies, "We Aussies like our fun, don't we, Clive?"

Clive, a handsome man with spiky, coal black hair and stylish upside-down glasses, turns uncertainly to his wife Laura, a painter with an ample figure and frizzy hair. She replies firmly, "You got that right, mate."

"Like Malouf says," Hal interjects, "it's the spirit of play."

"So, Louis, what do you do when you're at work?" I ask.

Louis is a beige-colored man with a receding, horseshoe-shaped hairline and a scholarly appearance. "I'm in construction."

I scan his short fingers, which seem soft. "What do you build?"

"Cement foundations, mostly."

His wife Emily, noticing my assessment of Louis' hands, explains, "He owns a company that builds foundations for commercial buildings in the Central Business District." Emily is a slender, elegant woman with long dark amber hair and heavy gold jewelry. She adds, "And I take care of our daughters. The youngest is only five, and she doesn't like me to leave."

"You should have had boys," Laura says with a laugh. "They always liked it when we left, and now *they've* left."

"Your boys are older," Emily replies. "That's different, isn't it?"

"It iss eassier to leave a baby," Dutchy says. "They don't complain."

Emily pales at this pragmatism. I don't know her any better than any of Reggie's other university friends who are gathered around this pub table, but I recognize Emily's maternal anxiety. To distract her from it, I say, "I see a construct of an Australian right at the table. I've never known a group this diverse who stayed connected for so many years." I raise my glass of wine and say, "To mateship!"

All but Joe and Graeme join me in the toast. Joe, who is sitting opposite, has drunk more than anyone and is sinking silently into despondence. He stares at his glass, occasionally fixing one of us with a glower. Graeme is seated beside Laura, his face set in a slight smile. He shows little and says less, and yet his manner is calm and open; I have difficulty paying heed to anyone else. He appears to ignore Reggie, but when her glass is empty, he fills it. Together, they form the table's center of gravity. He is strong and charismatic like her, but detached and cool. He seems to penetrate my being with his mind in a way that feels male but not sexual, patriarchal but not domineering. I expect others to notice his calm, intense presence, but they take him for granted.

It is Joe, oddly enough, who finally pinpoints Graeme's differentness by asking, "So how's the guru scam going?" Joe apparently means this to be funny, but it comes off like an aggrieved complaint. "You still wearing those fancy robes? And playing God as if you had all the answers?"

"Get stuffed," Roger remarks casually.

Roger's remark only encourages Joe, who continues, "You're the yellow-and red-robed, barefoot choir boy, aren't you Graeme?"

I am out of my depth among these long-time mates, who are rich and poor, polished and rough, esteemed and ignored, but I am beginning to be able to read them. While each seems kindly disposed to me for Reggie's sake, they are deeply distressed by Joe. I consider him carefully. He is in a bad way, but not bad looking. He would be attractive if he gave up petulant resentment, sat up straight, and rested easily in his chair instead of slouching over his folded arms. I entertain an impulse to take him on as a project, to see whether I can do for him what I couldn't do for Steve. I don't see how he'd be worse off. I decide to encourage him, perhaps even to offer him a little pity sex. I lean forward and show my cleavage. He doesn't respond. I reach out and touch his hand. I may be testing my feminine powers, or I may be drunk.

Reggie says pointedly, "Collo, come help me at the bar."

I have been ignoring the table, but now notice several empty glasses. I jump up and follow her to the bar, where she orders several pints. "You want to sleep with Joe, then, do you?"

"Well?" I say in confusion and embarrassment. "I suppose I was thinking that I might as well be kind. I'm single now, and I'm bound to sleep with someone, sometime."

"Let's walk."

We put the pints on the table, and then Reggie leads the way out the front door and down the steps into the cool night. We dodge the traffic whizzing along St. Kilda's Esplanade and stand at the low cement wall overlooking Port Phillip Bay. Behind us, tires squeal and horns honk. Ahead of us, the invisible, still air rests on the dark waters off Melbourne's shore.

"Is Graeme really a guru?"

"He has some students, some followers. He's careful not to push them too far or too fast. And he helps them stay out of trouble. I'd like to do the same for you."

I press the heels of my palms on the cold, rough wall and gaze intently into the darkness of sky and water. My mind's eye projects on it images of Steve and Joe side by side.

"Women here seem to be strong enough to give it away."

"We wouldn't give it to someone who turns everything into nothing."

"Like Joe?"

17

"Yes. You can't be kind without being strong. And when you're strong, you don't repeat your mistakes. Giving yourself to Joe would be like giving Shakespeare's canon to an illiterate. He wouldn't see your strengths or know how to appreciate or enhance them. And that's like giving yourself to Steve, isn't it?"

I take in a ragged breath. A braid of thoughts and feelings unwinds in my body. Steven and I confused masculinity with domination and femininity with submission. I thought he'd get stronger when I let him have his way. But he just got weaker and weaker.

"Right-o," Reggie continues. "You want you and your partner to synergize, to strengthen each other."

"To go from strength to strength."

"Yes."

As we turn back toward the Espy, my crown is several inches higher than it was when we started. I am poised to find a better partner. When I first came here, I saw St. Kilda as an urban jungle; now I see the wilds within.

By the time Reggie and I have made our way up the stoop and back inside to the table, Hal and Dutchy are gone, Roger is blowing smoke at Joe, and Joe is glowering at Rog. I surmise that Roger has teased Joe that I might have been interested in him and that Reggie has intervened. As she and I take our seats and prepare to enjoy our pints, Joe vents his anger on Graeme with a slurred insult.

Louis says firmly, "That's enough, Joe."

I catch Reggie's eye and mouth the words, "Thank you."

Reggie smiles slightly and asks Joe, "Why don't you come out with us more often?"

Joe's resentment collapses into self-pity. "I can't get all the way out here, can I? I don't have a car like you lot."

"You could take the train, Joe," Laura points out.

Louis and Emily leave shortly afterwards, followed by Joe trailing bitter curses. If he had Reggie's strength or Roger's guile, Joe could harm the group, and they would have to change him or exclude him. As it is, he is an irritant, a warning that virtues can be lost, and that their loss can negate prior accomplishments. When Laura and Clive stand to leave, the rest of us follow them outside into the still night.

After we part company with her friends, Reg and I take a long slow walk down the foreshore while talking about spiritual practice. I tell her of my Quaker and other radical Protestant forms of faith and practice, ones that support purposeful humanitarian change. She reminds me of her time in an ashram, and the peripatetic journeys that preceded her solo sailing and the journey up the coast of North America where we met.

"You know," I say, "we're almost complementary. Our explorations of being, becoming, and doing are broad but barely overlap."

"We could learn a lot from each other."

"It's an exciting prospect, isn't it? East and West are finally meeting—again, like two millenia ago when Jesus was a tantric master, like those gurus in India."

"Tantra is what I practice! But wait—" Reggie looks at her sailing watch. "It's time we met my mates Liz and Ronnie."

We plunge into the urban jungle of St Kilda, suspending our lifelong conversation on change for the present.

3
Pub Crawl

I t is dark now, but the air is still hair-dryer hot. At the corner of Fitzroy and Grey, bright lights illuminate enchanted faces waiting for a green light. People continue to arrive from trams, from Luna Park carnival rides, and from the palm-lined beach below. A bead of sweat runs down my back; I wish us back at the shore, which was cooler.

The light seems stuck on red. An ancient green and yellow tram is rolling into the intersection, blocking traffic, and raising a chorus of metallic complaints. When the tram clears the corner, cars that had been trapped behind it leap away like greyhounds after a mechanical hare. On our left, a trio of drunken carousers leans into the slipstream as if reaching for a bride's bouquet. Behind us, a sour-smelling man in a Hawaiian shirt props up his wilted date and tells her dreamily that the Southern Ocean winds will soon sweep up and push this summer scorcher up into the Outback.

I glance at Reggie. Her faint smile and vivid denim eyes shine with characteristic serenity and joy. She seems a center of calm as always, though tonight she appears unusually elegant in a slip dress of midnight blue, shiny sandals, and a loose topknot of hennaed hair. Her presence feels a head taller than the rest of us. I too, am dressed up; I have shed my old skin of overalls, head kerchief, and long braid to put chopsticks in my updo and to wear the jacaranda-blue nightgown that we are all pretending is a dress.

A voice bawls out, "This place is too bloody posh!"

Another whoops, "It's wankers only!"

The screamers run at us from the brightly lit mouth of the George Hotel across the street. One is wearing heavy red lipstick, a smeared beauty mark, and a black dress stretched tightly over large hips. The other is in hoop earrings, bright pink lipstick, and a shiny white miniskirt that tops her gangly legs. The pair splash through the stream of traffic, narrowly missing an orange Japanese motorcycle, a red Lamborghini, and an old blue Holden with a hailstorm's worth of dents. I recognize them with a shock: they are the childhood "mates" I've seen in photographs.

The large woman vaults the curb and halts nose-to-nose with Reggie to snarl, "Those pouncey prats can get stuffed! I don't care if they buy your wine. We want to go to a pub with real blokes!"

"Dinky di jackaroos!" the skinny one shrieks.

I can't believe these are Liz and Ronnie, but I am not surprised that their abuse disappears into Reggie and boomerangs back as endearments. She puts a palm on the big one's shoulder and says tenderly, "You're done here, then, are you Ronnie? Shall we do a pub crawl?"

Veronica's expression crumples. "Yeah. A pub crawl."

The skinny one hoots, "Ronnie's desperate for a root!"

"I just wanted a nice night. You know how much I need a nice night." A tear streaks black kohl down Veronica's right cheek. The streetlight turns green. The crowd in front of us pours away. The four of us remain like trees parting a herd of cattle.

"Right-o, Ronnie." Reggie holds out a packet of pocket handkerchiefs.

Veronica takes a tissue. As she rubs her lower eyelid, her eyes light on me, and her face contorts. She confronts me like a saltwater crocodile protecting its nest. "What are you staring at?"

"This is my friend Colette Connolly from the States. Colette, these are my mates, Ronnie and Liz."

Reggie pivots smartly and strides up Grey Street. I try to catch up, but Veronica blocks me adroitly. I fall back with Liz, wishing I knew how to translate my manners and mores into Australian ones.

"Collo'll be working for Grandma and me," Reggie says pleasantly to Veronica. "And with Andy as well."

"Andy's scone hot!" Liz cackles.

We pass a Salvation Army shelter for battered women. Across the street, unlicensed sex workers lurk in a row of bushes like a many-legged demon wearing thigh-high boots, heels, and cheap slippers. I remember Sister Adrian's disciplinary ruler, which taught generations of us schoolgirls that women could only become devilish temptresses or celibate sourpusses. My palm smarts as I remember that I will be facing hard choices about my sexuality.

As we walk, Liz patters like a guide with a repertoire of one-liners. When she spots the commercial sex workers she says, "They'd get more clients if they went starkers."

When we pass the Sacred Heart Mission, she says, "It's too quiet here. Bet all the blokes are down at the Daily Planet brothel!"

By the time we take our next turn, Liz's gaiety has become a welcome flavor in the intoxicating cocktail of Australia, a cocktail sweetened with Reggie's happiness and salted with the island nation's myths of the Dreamtime, stories of exiled convicts, and memories of Jewish, Greek, and Italian shopkeepers who escaped war-torn Europe. All of these flavor my sanguine—or insane—search for a new life.

A block on, I feel comfortable enough to venture, "How about a café? I've drunk too much liquor already."

Veronica wheels around and spits, "Any two-pot screamer can bloody well go home!"

"You can order a soda, if you like," Reggie suggests mildly.

We continue past blocks of flats that rise like human rookeries; low Edwardian homes that recall a wave of suburban optimism; and signs of new affluence, like fenced-in construction sites and double storefronts displaying rusty tools next to upscale baby clothes. In this economic intertidal zone, we are all poised to ride a rising tide of fortune.

As we approach the open door of a pub, Reggie slows. On the façade above the door, large green Canterbury letters announce, "The Duke Hotel." A line of men dressed in jeans and work shoes extends from the door like mutineers on a gangplank. Rows of grimy multi-paned windows with frilly tie-back curtains bracket the door. Above them, the pub rises like a beached schooner with square portholes. I mutter, "Mutton dressed as lamb."

Liz shoots me a keen glance. She is sharper than she lets on.

"I mean the sweet curtains. And me, I suppose."

Reggie strides inside and Liz follows, but Veronica lingers to lean into a tall, hook-nosed man with wild growths of ear hairs. She asks in a throaty voice, "Fancy a bit of the amber fluid?"

He steps back, looks away, and shakes his head. She glowers and plunges inside.

One of the others murmurs wistfully, "She looks cheap, mate."

"Ah, you never know 'til you wake up. Last one cleaned out my pockets."

"I'd risk it for the redhead," adds a third with careless menace.

I dart inside, relieved to find the interior well-lit and homey. The décor is down-home gumbo, with a carefully kept wall shrine to the St. Kilda Saints Aussie Rules football club which displays historic photos and red, white, and black guernseys. An ill-kept snooker table with blotchy red felt peeks out through a crumbling arch on the left.

I join Reggie and Liz at the wallaby-colored bar, where a publican is pulling pints for a blond man with beefy, freckled thighs. Ronnie lights a cigarette and surveys the room with a scowl, venting her frustration by asking me to choose a table and then rejecting each of my choices. She soon tires of it and takes a seat. I join her and follow her eyes around the room, noting the early starters who have become groggy or grim-faced. One is resting his head on his arm, behind his mug, which makes his eyes bug out like a bee's. Liz brings two brown stubbies to the table. Ronnie downs half a bottle and starts gossiping in Liz's ear.

Reggie arrives and hands me a petite pot of beer.

"Thanks! So, is this like a bar that bans open-toed shoes?"

"Ay?"

"You know, a guy place that wants to exclude women but can't, for legal reasons."

"Ah, look, there are probably a few women in the ladies' saloon." She raises her pot toward a back passageway, where I see a curtained doorway to a side room. "Newer pubs don't have those, but this one's been here for yonks. There's still a jasmine-covered dunny out back."

"An outhouse? Really?"

"They kitted it out with toilets and sinks, but it's a dunny all the same."

"How do they fit a sink into a dunny?"

"Stupid question," Ronnie observes blandly, stubbing out her smoke on the shiny wooden tabletop.

"I'll show you!" Liz giggles, and hops out of her seat. She leads the way past the ladies' saloon, where a few couples are cuddling, and into a back passage that smells of beer and soap-shunning men. She exits a rear door and crosses a small grassy yard to a brick outbuilding with three narrow white doors, and pushes open the middle one to point to a teapot-sized sink stuck onto the side wall.

"Very economical use of space. Very bad smell."

Liz giggles amiably. I return to the back door and hold it open for a wiry man with a graying ponytail who exits as I enter. Halfway up the back passage, I turn back to look for Liz and see her standing with her hand on the man's crotch. For a moment, I am transfixed by her reckless boldness, and then recover my wits and dart back to the table. I take a swig of hops-heavy brew and think of knitting in my favorite easy chair back in Maine. I feel a bit like an ex-con longing for lockdown.

"Where's Liz?" Veronica demands.

I raise my eyebrows and stare at a bubble gathering at the bottom of my tiny glass pot. Ronnie stands huffily, stubs her cigarette, and stomps to the back. She returns with the giddily grinning Liz. When they sit down, Ronnie glowers at Liz and fumes, "I can't believe you went after him! I wanted him!"

"I got a pash off him!" Liz declares.

I picture them kissing passionately and regret it immediately. When the pony-tailed man returns, Liz takes a lipstick out of her purse, colors her lips slowly, and smacks them theatrically. Veronica settles into a sulk. She finishes a second stubby and starts another.

"So, you've been here before?" I ask Reggie.

"Reg used to come here with me, didn't you Reg?" Veronica interjects.

"Ah, yeah. It's the kind of place that serves its suburb well. Never trendy, never empty."

"It reminds me of my father," I say.

"What, never trendy?"

I laugh. "No! He'd go to a bar like this now and then and tie one on, and then we'd have to hide from him when he came home."

Veronica looks at me like a television program she loves to hate.

"A boozer!" Liz giggles.

"He was an angry drunk, was he?" Reggie asks with concern.

Veronica trains her eyes on me like a film critic making a list of complaints. Liz takes advantage of Ronnie's distraction to catch the eye of the man with the ponytail.

"No, I had a very happy childhood. He and mom were good to us and loved each other like crazy. But he was a typical postwar factory worker: A good worker and a binger."

The man with the ponytail gets up and disappears into the back. Liz follows. Veronica doesn't notice because she is watching me the way a cat watches a bird.

"I didn't know he worked in a factory. I thought Peoria was rural," Reg notes.

"The manufacturing is all but gone now, but back then it had a strong industrial base."

"Like the north of England."

"Exactly."

"What was your old man's job?" Veronica asks neutrally, blowing a cloud of smoke to the side.

"He worked in tool and die."

"What's that?"

"It's making the machines that make machines. He started out cutting metal and worked his way up to foreman."

"Hah!" Veronica is finally ready to pounce. "He was a bloody manager!"

I glance ruefully at Reggie. As I open my mouth to apologize for precipitating an insult, Veronica continues, "Don't look at Reg! She makes a bloody living work of art, doesn't she?"

"Yes, yes she does," I say, suppressing a smile.

Veronica runs down my father. I am transported back to Sunday morning Mass, when the hard discipline of sitting still constricted my ribs like an outgrown dress.

When Veronica starts in on expats, I realize I'm playing with my wedding band, and stare at it in astonishment. I had forgotten it. I pull it off and drop it into my purse, baring a stripe of pale skin. When I look up, Reggie's face offers concern. I try to smile reassurance, but worry about the future.

When Liz returns with an expression of casual triumph, Veronica realizes that she has been had. She pushes her breasts out like two chunks of cheese in a rattrap and scans the room again. When she spots a bulky man with a shaven head, thick neck, and elaborate tattoo sleeves, she waves at him. When he heaves to his feet and plods stuporously toward the back, she follows him. After a time too short for credibility, she returns with a pasted-on smile and says, "What a pash!"

Liz pipes at me, "You'd be happy, too, if you got a pash off Andy!"

"I'm off men for now, thanks."

This only encourages Liz. She teases me until my face is as red as a sunburned tourist on St. Kilda beach. When the tattooed man stumbles back to his seat, Veronica stops feigning interest in Liz's teasing and twists around to catch his eye. Reggie tries to turn our attention to the plans for our weekend outing to her mother's beach house, but Ronnie is determined. When the man sees her, he stares at us with an expression that could equally signal desire or rage. His brows slowly contract in a samurai frown. My heart sinks.

"Ronnie fancies the Hulk!" Liz hoots.

Beside the Hulk sits a tall, menacing man with high cheekbones, bulging arms, and a shaved head. He looks at the Hulk and then at us, and grabs the Hulk's forearm. The Hulk grimaces, makes a fist with his free hand, and moves it back like a pitcher preparing to throw a sinker. He moves the fist forward slowly, like a certified fight instructor teaching an actor how to look as if he is fighting. While the fist is in the air, I hope that he is only pretending to throw the punch, but when it strikes the tall man's cheek it leaves a cut that dribbles blood.

The men seated at neighboring tables rise, circle the brawlers, and watch them rise and embrace like heavyweight toddlers. They are too angry to avoid a pointless fight or to foresee its miserable consequences. Their muscles swell and sharpen. Grunts rumble from their bellies. For a moment, they totter like a dance couple, and then seem to freeze at an angle that defies gravity.

Finally, the tall man falls back onto a table that tips and drops a dozen bottles and glasses to the floor. Some break. The Hulk seizes the tall man's shoulders and pitches him in our direction. We jump up and scatter as the tall man falls on our table. Before the Hulk's fist can connect again, the tall man grabs the Hulk's tattooed arm and pulls. The Hulk turns, loses his balance, and falls on top of the tall man. The legs of our table snap. The top crashes onto the carpet of broken glass. Both men fall on top of it.

The impact rattles my heels and rouses the stony spectators. When the Hulk winds up again, several men grab and pin his arms. Others close in until the brawl is a scrum that moves, amoeba-like, between the tables toward the front door. When it exits, the formation breaks and the brawlers tumble out onto the sidewalk. Reggie and I go to a front window, from which we see the tall man stagger away. A few men pull the Hulk to his feet and tamp him into the back of a small car that rolls away down the street.

I hear Veronica crow, "Did you see the way they fought over me?"

Dumbfounded, I turn to search her face for signs of recognition that either man might have killed the other, accidentally or on purpose. A skull might have cracked against the edge of a chair, or a throat might have been torn out by broken glass. Either could have held his anger, followed us, and raped or killed one of us. Ronnie's face shows no sign that any such harsh possibility has occurred to her. I look to Reggie for guidance and see that she is unsurprised but sad.

"He wanted a bash-up more than he wanted a root!" Liz hoots.

"Did you see that, Reg? They fought over me!" Veronica repeats. She turns to me and says with pity, "Bet you wish they'd wanted you!"

Ronnie is trying to include me. I do my best to assemble my features into an expression of concord. She and Reggie and I lift the remains of the broken table while Liz snatches her crushed purse, and we walk to the back yard and set the wooden pieces against a fence. The energy of the fight must have formed a bond between us; we dawdle like an elderly lawn bowls team after a match, until Ronnie leads us to the front door, solicitously pointing out bits of broken glass and a posse of angry men that wants free pints to replace those they lost in the brawl. When we regain the cooling air of Barkly Street and have walked a full block in silence, I venture, "I don't understand that kind of fighting."

"They're men, aren't they? That's what they do," Ronnie replies helpfully.

"Think with their cocks!" Liz cackles.

"TGIF. Time for a pub-crawl and brawl," I say to Liz.

"I reckon the bald one had a bad hair day," Reggie says with a sly smile.

"A dust-up a day keeps the women at bay," I continue.

"A hit in time saves nine."

As Reggie and I trade inanities, Liz and Ronnie walk briskly ahead of us, apparently embarrassed. I giggle when they distance themselves to keep up social standards that I don't recognize. By the time we reach the next pool of streetlight, I am giddy. I feel buoyant. Realizing it, I stop abruptly; my mouth opens in an "O" of astonishment. *This can't be happening. My mood is too good to be true.* Back in Maine, I would have taken an hour or a day to recover from a lack of perfect consensus; here, I recovered within minutes from the shock of a violent exchange.

I glance at Reggie and see her habitual benignant smile topped by raised eyebrows that question my pause. My resilience is coming from her. A still voice whispers in my heart, *This joy is hers.* I resume moving, slowly, looking ahead on the street and back on my first week down under. Beneath the superficial rush of jet lag and logistics is a profound uprooting. I haven't understood my impulse to leave the old life or to come all the way to this island continent. I am lucky that Reggie is helping me through it.

Reggie remarks casually, as if continuing a conversation, "You were right about avoiding alcohol. I shouldn't drive tonight. Let's stay at Mum's and drive down to Blairgowrie in the morning. When we come back, we'll meet up with Andy and finish stocking up on supplies."

"Sounds good. But isn't your mother—Anne, isn't it—coming back here this weekend?"

"Mid-week. We'll be out by then."

A tram passes. A somber-eyed girl peers out of the front window like Gretel in a forest comprised of over-talking teens, old women with shopping trolleys, and sorry-looking couples heading for Balaclava. When I know that my voice will not be lost in the tram's tired clanking, I ask, "Tell me, why are you friends with them? Ronnie's resentment is exhausting."

"Puts you off, does she?"

"I could never deal with her on my own."

"Ah, look, she suffers from negativities. But we needn't react."

"You mean take what she dishes out?" I ask.

"Not at all. It can be a work of a lifetime, or of many lifetimes, but you can choose to *not* mirror others. I'm half way there; I can transform those kinds of feelings with friends, but I can't do it with family."

"How do you do that with friends?"

Reggie pauses, and then says slowly, "You mentioned tantra before. I use it continuously. It's the ultimate fruit of late classical Indian civilization, a fundamental practice for constant change that is redemptive. You can use it to turn hate into love, fear into courage, greed into generosity, deathly thoughts into life-giving ones."

"So … you change your own bad habits into good ones, and those who love you may change with you?"

"It starts out that way. If you keep it up, you can work to change the world from the inside out."

"What do you do, exactly? I've done inner and outer work, but not like that!"

"I'll try to explain. The classic teachings use the metaphor of hand-weaving a rug, but most people don't know how to weave," Reggie replies thoughtfully.

"I do! You saw my loom and my tapestries back at the farm in Maine."

"Right, then. As an artist, you could probably come up with many other metaphors, but let's stick with the weaving."

"Works for me."

"Think of something you do continuously, like breathing. Imagine you were graphing it one second at a time."

"Like making a dotted, sinuous line?" I ask.

"Yes. One that begins at birth and continues until death. Let's call it a living process, and think of it as one of the warp threads of the tapestry of your life."

"So, one of the long and strong and often hidden threads that hold the decorative cross-threads of the rug's pattern."

"Exactly. Now imagine that every living process that you could graph in time is forming one of the warp threads of your life—everything you do continuously, in stillness, motion, or action."

"That's a lot of warp threads."

"Imagine that they're thinner than hairs, and that you're creating a tapestry in time while you're walking. Think of it as like the imprint you leave in the air, or the wake you leave in water."

"I can't picture something that fluid and multidimensional— not on the fly, at any rate. I'll stick with the rug metaphor, thank you."

"Good idea; easy to visualize. So now, let's say that you don't like one of your processes. Maybe you are still angry at a nun you haven't seen for twenty years, for example," Reggie says slyly.

"You know I am. And yes, I know it's like taking poison and waiting for someone else to die!"

"So in tantra, you let the thread break and you don't pick it up. A community of people with similar threads could do it together."

"How?"

"Let's wait on that until we've established the metaphor."

"I think I have it. You keep the good habit threads, drop the bad ones, and add in better ones."

"Yes, and you do it gradually for stability."

"Right: If a whole community did what I just did—broke a lot of threads at once—it could fall apart. Like I might have done if you hadn't taken me in!"

"I want to take up some of yours, ones that can model change from the outside in, like peacemaking."

"We could teach each other! I would dearly love to get on with Ronnie."

"You're already doing that."

"Not entirely." I sigh. "Tonight upset me because of the particular darkness around Liz and Ronnie's sexuality. When men disparage and—well, hate, really—women's sexuality and degrade it and—" I have to stop and breathe to keep my cool. When I'm calmer, I continue. "So I find it distressing to see women degrade themselves. Especially Ronnie, because she can't see the harm she does. To all of us."

"Let's look at it as an opportunity. The profane is the raw material of the sacred. When she recognizes something better, she can choose—assuming she agrees that moving sexuality away from the profane is a good thing."

"As I do," I say.

"Tantra has a lot of sexual practices that are good for that. Would you like me to teach you some simple ones this weekend?"

"Me?"

"You and Liz and Ronnie. It'll give them more choices. Might give you some as well. Be good for all of us."

"Together?" I ask warily.

"You can have as much privacy as you like. But you'll want me around in case things come up that upset you. Body work can do that."

"I'm not sure that's for me."

"Wouldn't want to leave those patterns as is."

"What do you mean?"

"Better to let the dark bits go. Free up your body for—what did you call it? The joy?"

"The secret of joy. I knew there'd be a catch."

"Probably a minor one. But you never know."

I laugh. "This officially makes my first week down under the strangest of my life! I understand less and less about Australia every day. I thought I got it when you told me about it, and then when I stepped off the plane, and then when I stayed here in St. Kilda. But I was like a traveler seeing it through tips in a guidebook, and now you've taken it global!"

"So. How are you liking it so far?" Reggie asks seriously.

"It's the adventure of a lifetime. Aussies and Americans speak English and shop at the same chain stores, but I'm beginning to see that our similarities are superficial. Our differences are deep, and mysterious, and intriguing. I want to figure them out, and when I do I'll—I'll—"

"Be ready to move on?"

"Be somebody new," I say with wonder.

4

Yin Rising

As we approach the neighborhood of Brunswick, where Reggie's father started his first restaurant and where Liz and Ronnie still live, I idly wish that we wouldn't stop to pick them up. But when we see them standing side by side at the curb, their faces radiant, flowery beach bags at their sides, I am happy to see them, and to have the chance to know them away from dark urban nights that defy illumination. They seem happy to see me, too, and I am gratified to think that we are no longer strangers. Little do I suspect that this will be an eventful day, or that we will be mates by the end of it.

As Reggie drives us south along Port Phillip Bay, which rests on our right like a giant bowl of blue-green jelly, we chat about our ups and downs, sharing caricatures of those who have thwarted us. We exit the road at a teahouse that is tucked between the road and a wooded park. We stand in line with a small luncheon crowd to order fish and chips and sweet black tea, and, after our order is ready, take our food trays to a table on the back deck. We eat slowly, enjoying the thickets of trees that shelter us from the sun and wind, and offer glimpses of distant children playing in the procession of whitecaps that is climbing the beach of an adjacent marine reserve.

As we finish our tea, a lone barefoot boy in a wet T-shirt

comes running at us; he stops on the other side of the railing to stare at me. After listening a minute, he pokes his head under the top rail and says to me, "Say candy!"

"What's that?"

Liz pipes up, "Say candy for him!"

"Okay. Candy!"

He laughs. His belly moves in and out like the breast of a bird. "Say it again!"

I repeat it several times. In the near distance, a woman gripping a wriggling toddler calls him to her. As he runs reluctantly away, I ask Liz, "What was that about?"

"We say lolly," Veronica explains.

Ronnie and Liz take turns sharing their favorite Australianisms, or strine. I learn that swimsuits are bathers, suntan lotion is suncream, a chat is a natter, a fight is a bash-up, and so on. After tiring of the vernacular, and then exhausting the topic of lipstick colors, Veronica orders a pint and turns to her favorite topic. "The Queen can dissolve our government anytime she pleases! She did it to Gough Whitlam and she'll do it again. We need a bloody constitution."

"What happened?"

Reggie explains, "When Gough Whitlam was Prime Minister, the Governor General called elections, and even put the army on alert."

"Whitlam stuffed it up!" Liz says.

"He bloody well did, but the Queen shouldn't be able to sack him, should she? It's none of her bizzo. We should have a Republic, unless we can have Wills."

I see a problem with her logic, but am happy to ignore it.

Ronnie continues, "Diana was the only one who understood

the job. The Queen can't even buy herself a dress."

"I fancy Fergie!" Liz giggles. "It's those toes!"

Back in the car, Ronnie and Liz return to the back seat together to devour a stack of pulp magazines. Reggie drives south on the inside shore of the Mornington Peninsula, rolling down her window to let a cool breeze tousle her hair. I lean on my elbow and get lost in memories. The onshore breeze brings whiffs of salty decay from the sea's edge that remind me of the smell of the Atlantic off the coast of Maine. I watch the water and relive childhood trips to the Wisconsin lakeshores where I first exposed my body to the sun and—in spite of taboos instilled by priests and parents—allowed my flesh to teach me of sensual relaxation and of the urge for sexual expression. I daydream a mishmash of beaches and barns in a jumble of rural Maine and Melbourne.

Abruptly, I realize that Reggie has been talking to me. "Did you say something?"

Reggie smiles cryptically. "You're ready for the beach, then, are you?"

"Can't wait to do what my friends and family probably think I'm doing."

Reggie makes an equivocal sound as the road leaves the shore and passes through the long stretch of tarmac-dead strip malls that line the road through Dromana. There, she turns back toward the Bay and heads west through a series of long, narrow beach towns that remind me of the Great Lakes. These, though, extend from the calm, warm waters of Port Phillip Bay on our right to the rough, cold waters of Bass Strait beyond the low rise on our left.

We pass by a long windbreak that separates the road from the Bay's beach. Reggie slows before we reach the resort town of Blairgowrie and turns left on a wooded road. She enters a tidy, tree-rich suburb and veers suddenly right into a circular drive. She stops the car in front of a modest, one-story ranch house that has the same 1950s style and mature garden of trees and shrubs as the others around it. Reggie cuts the motor. We step out of our warm seats into a cooling breeze bearing birdsong and the perfume of hidden flowers.

Reggie goes to open the front screen door, rummaging in her dangling shoulder purse for her keys to the beach house. She finds them and opens the locked and shuttered house. We enter a large front room that seems like a time capsule from my childhood with its large picture windows, wood-paneled walls, and a breakfast bar that separates the dining area from an L-shaped kitchenette in the far corner. On a low table surrounded by a mid-century sofa and chairs sits a tiny black-and-white television set with rabbit-ear antennae. Beyond the kitchen, a hall leads back to three bedrooms, a bath, a toilet, and a door to the back yard. Over the kitchen sink is a window through which we can see the big golden brick barbecue in the back.

The air inside smells of Reggie's mother Anne's best-loved blooms, and the baskets on the floor and countertops are filled with groceries, toiletries, and upscale glossy magazines. Cozy familiarity envelops and eases us.

"This is so homey!"

"Make yourselves at home then, ladies," Reggie says, disappearing into the toilet at the back.

Liz and Ronnie go to a back bedroom with two single beds and plop their bags down to unpack. I put Reggie's bags and mine in the bedroom opposite and hang our towels in the bath. Liz, Ronnie, and Reggie turn on the utilities, inventory the cupboards, make tea, and plan a dinner. Without saying a word, they fall into a smooth and efficient workflow. At first I take their cooperation as a sign that they have opened the cottage before, but soon realize that they, like Andy, find it natural to work as a team. I cannot enter the flow as easily.

Before I can identify a useful task, Reggie and Ronnie leave to buy fresh meats and produce for a barbecue, and Liz tells me to get ready to go with her to the beach. We put on sunhats and bathers and go on a pet's tour of the neighborhood, beginning at the mailbox post beside the front drive and continuing along a roadside strip of sandy soil. We pass by a grouping of annuals in a neighboring garden, pause at the fire hydrant at the end of the block, and at the highway dash across the tarmac and through a thicket of stunted ironbark trees. We emerge abruptly to a wide, flat, sandy shore that extends along the brackish bay in both directions for as far as we can see.

I whoop and run with my arms out like a child playing airplane, enjoying the freedom and expansiveness of the seemingly endless sand. Liz laughs; we are both content. After splashing through the still, warm water near the shore, we turn west and walk above the tidal line on damp hard-packed sand where our feet leave no prints. When Liz finds a dry spot to her liking, she stops and sits. I plop beside her on the seaweed-laced sand and gaze out on the smooth, silvery waters of the Bay. We laze and watch the pale yellow sun slowly decline toward a gray, cloud-streaked horizon.

"Liz, are there sharks in the Bay?"

"Not as such." The correct answer, I find out later, is rarely.

"Are there poisonous redback spiders or big brown snakes around here?"

"I want to see a Tazzie Tiger!"

Eventually, I stop expecting conversation and join in idle natter. When we spot a tiny woman with a Jack Russell terrier straining at his leash, I ask, "Who's walking whom?"

Liz giggles. When a man with an enormous beer belly plods by pulling a distractible Welsh Corgi, she says, "He's desperate for a dunny!"

We walk west and pass a widely-spaced row of bathing boxes. Some are closed; those that are open spill out wine-drinking couples or picnicking families onto the sand like dice from over-turned shakers. When the orange sun-fire dims to an ember, and the water and sky glisten like a sheet of tarnishing silver, we turn back and retrace our steps past the boxes, this time greeting some folks like old neighbors.

Before darkness overtakes us, we dash up the beach, across the highway, and up to the house, where we find Reggie and Ronnie grilling chicken in the back yard. Liz and I go into the kitchen to make salads. As night thickens, we say less and less; we eat quietly, in a way that is languorous and satisfying. At nine o'clock, when we are done lingering over the last tidbits of fruit and cheese, we move as one to clean up. I wash dishes so that the others have to fit in with me. In half an hour, I am lounging in a green tweed armchair in the front room, thumbing through a glossy magazine dedicated to Australian country living.

At 9:30, the screen door snaps shut and Veronica and Liz race past me in the direction of their bedroom, where they make slumber-party sounds of muffled laughs, whispers, scraping zippers, and closing drawers. I wonder momentarily if they are planning a skinny dip and then get lost in a photo of a cabin in the Blue Mountains. Sometime later, I hear couch springs creak and peel my eyes away from an herb garden fantasy to find Reggie sitting on the couch, looking at me expectantly. I wonder what I missed.

"Collo, are you ready for the teaching?"

I tense up, try to force my body to relax, and then give up. "As ready as I'll ever be," I say, closing my magazine.

Since leaving my marriage behind, I have felt nothing but relief—until this moment. Reg has been asking, "Has it hit you yet?" It hits me now. I am transported back in time to Maine. I recall Steve's face contorting with spite as he says, "Practice makes perfect—bullshit—you'll never get any better at it!" After a time, I look up at Reggie. She is waiting patiently, a kindly expression on her face. *This isn't about me. It's about Liz and Ronnie.* I remember the bash-up at the pub. I remember how worried we were about them. Reggie is giving me a chance to engage myself in keeping them safe by offering them an alternative to anonymous sex. And she said it would be good for her, too.

"I have a question," I say hesitantly. "How would better sex keep Liz and Ronnie safe?"

Now Reggie looks confused. "Not better sex; more intentional. More theirs."

Inside my skin, an electric fence switches on, one cobbled together from a lifetime of tragicomic emotional overloads that enforced my childhood sexual taboos. It includes the cold Sunday when I am disgusted to see my brother Sean peek up the skirt of Melissa's dotted Swiss Easter dress; the moment when my hymen breaks, and I am convinced that sex is a humiliating and hurtful mistake; the time when Da makes me swear to be chaste so he won't have to disown me; and Sister Adrian's ruler stinging my palm as she struggles with lewd thoughts that she imagines are mine. I feel an intense desire to lose my fear of wagging tongues and social condemnation. I toss my magazine on the floor.

"And less profane?"

"And less susceptible to Andy."

My face flushes to my hairline. Reggie can read me like no other; I am pierced with embarrassment. My heart races; my breath goes shallow and spare.

"I feel your desire for Andy, and yet you've said you don't want to have sex with him—or with anyone. I can teach you to satisfy your desire or to quell it, so that it will be easy to want no and to say no. You could start tonight with a few simple practices, breathing techniques and such. "

"Breathing? Why breathing?"

"Breathing guides the flow of energy to channel it for ecstasy, or celibacy."

"Celibacy? Liz and Ronnie are considering celibacy?"

"No, but you might."

"I might! I was going to become a nun until I saw that it made people cruel."

"Choosing celibacy is entirely different to being forced into it."

"I don't want to become a sourpuss!"

"I think you'll find that an energy practice can lead to contented celibacy," Reggie says.

Liz and Ronnie emerge from the back bedroom with blanket rolls. Liz giggles and says to me, "We're going to have sex, want to *come?*"

Ronnie adds, "Come with us, and *come* all you want!"

Reggie says, "I'll join you two in the car straightaway."

Ronnie pokes Liz's arm, and they exit whispering and giggling. The screen door slams shut with a hollow thwack.

"I'll begin by teaching you to satisfy your needs on your own. If you decide to learn more later, I can teach you to turn sexual energy into relaxation, or happiness."

"May I ask… are you a lesbian like Steve says?"

"I hope I don't fit into any category. But I reckon not. Graeme is my partner and my consort—but please don't tell anyone. I know how the family will react, and I don't want to rock the boat while we're starting up the inn at Grandma's place. We'll have enough stress to cope with. But you met him, and you've noticed that he's also keen on transformation. He is the one who taught me the sexual practices."

"So did you ever have sex with a woman?"

"Ah, yeah, years ago. I was with a bloke who wanted two women, and we took a friend to bed. While I watched him with her, I saw he wasn't trying to please her, and realized he'd never bothered himself about me. I left him that night and started searching for something better. I became aware of the possibility of total fulfillment, physical, emotional—everything. And then I found Graeme, and we accelerated our transformation."

In the front drive, a horn honks.

"So, we'll be doing some kind of pagan ritual?"

"No. I invoke the sacred by saying something accessible, usually something Daoist about yin and yang, or a Gaia reference to Mother Earth and Father Sky. And then we work individually, in our own ways."

The word work pleases my inner Sister Adrian. "Work. And no ritual?"

"I'm no guru. Tantra used to be transmitted by initiation, but you can learn it with the help of a guide, which allows you to find your own path. It isn't as powerful, but it gives you a chance to search for something new."

"So, you would say a few words and then we would go masturbate alone?"

"I like to call it self-pleasuring with the possibility of meaning," Reggie replies. She stands and states firmly, "If you want to try, you'll have to organize a blanket and pillow. Liz and Ronnie are too keen to wait much longer!"

I jump up and run to the bedroom. When I return, Reggie hands me a small box. "Why don't you have a go with these *ben wa* balls? They're small and gentle and private. Liz and Ronnie won't know you have them in unless you tell them. And they're no good covered in sand. You'd best put them in here."

"Put them where?" I look around in confusion. Reggie raises an eyebrow; my face burns. "Okay, I got it. In my—listen, you could tell me to swallow them and I wouldn't know any better."

I retreat to the bedroom and open the sealed box. Inside, two small, dense, brassy spheres stare up like gilded eyeballs. I undress, take them from the red faux velvet folds in which they rest, lie back on the bed, and push them inside as far as possible. When I stand up, I can't feel them. I dress, wash my hands, and run out to the car, arguing with myself.

I'm telling you, it's no big deal.

It's the nuttiest thing you've ever done, bar none! What would Steve say?

Who cares? I want to be free of him. I want to be free of the fears of others.

When I get into the car Liz chirps, "I'll show you mine if you show me yours!" I turn around to see her holding up a vibrator with an attachment that looks like a scalp massager.

"Mine's bigger!" Ronnie quips. She holds up a huge purple dildo with rubbery appendages. She turns it on. It lights up and vibrates fiercely. The dangly bits squirm. "It's got great clit ticklers!"

"Show us yours, Collo!" Liz says.

"I can't! I'm wearing the *ben wa* balls!" I say boldly.

"Show us your balls, Collo!" Liz giggles.

"Don't make me laugh, Lizzie, I'll push them out!"

"You don't need gadgets if you take time to explore the peaks and valleys," Reggie says as she turns east along the ocean road.

"I reckon Collie's never had a valley!" Liz giggles.

"Who needs valleys?" Veronica retorts truculently. "I just want peaks."

I didn't think to tell Reggie that I grew up fearing masturbation. I would feel silly mentioning that now, or admitting that I have no idea what they mean by valleys. My psyche crashes against the cage bars that confine my sexuality; the impact shakes me awake. I see now that Ronnie and Liz are free of qualms, and that they have a kind of bold strength that I lack. I have more to learn than I know.

A mile or so on, Reggie pulls off the road, cuts the car motor, and shuts off the headlamps, leaving us in utter darkness. When we get out, onshore gusts whip our clothes. Reggie's flashlight marks the way over a field of uneven, matted grass. We wrap ourselves in blankets and follow her beam. As our eyes adjust, we see the moon, a few stars, and the silhouettes of twisted trees. Reggie's light passes through the trees and disappears.

What do you think you're doing?

I'm going down to the beach at night.

That's ridiculous! You're in way over your head already. How will you masturbate? You've never even tried it.

It must be easy or the nuns wouldn't have been afraid of it.

A hand grabs my arm. Liz's voice shouts, "We stop ahead and creep down."

Crashing surf and howling wind below us paint a sonic

picture of a bluff beyond a windbreak. We soon see moonlight touching the foamy crests of the twelve-foot waves that pound a steep, narrow beach beyond the bluff. This is nothing like the peaceful bay on the other side of the peninsula. The scene is disorienting, like a rite of initiation, or a hazing, or a wilder Aussie view of risk.

Reggie's beam descends diagonally below the edge of the bluff. In the lulls between crashing waves, we hear her steps cascade pebbles down the steep trail. I can't see her or the others, but I manage to overcome my fear by leaning into the bluff with my elbow and feeling my way with my feet. I am more confident now: I have done something unexpected. Something risky. The rest will be easier.

When my feet touch down on the sand, I see Liz's silhouette following the zigzag beam of Reggie's flashlight, and I follow her in turn toward the luminescent backdrop of the high surf. The beam shows a glimpse of Ronnie putting her bundle several yards above the foam. I do the same. Hands take mine and lift them high above my head. I hear Reggie's voice shout, "We offer the yin of the earth to the yang of the heavens. We fill our physical bodies with life energy and let it flow into our energy bodies, and then into our spiritual bodies, and then into the Dao. May our ecstasy unite the earth with the sky, the temporal with the eternal."

I suppress a nervous laugh. I see a cartoon in my head of a coven of crazies intent on making love to the Southern Crux, the Aussie counterpart of the North Star.

How silly can you get?

Abruptly, the circle breaks and I am alone in the dark, feeling the sound and pull of a powerful riptide that is racing away into the Southern Ocean.

I pick up my blanket roll and feel my way back to and along the bottom of the bluff. Ten paces on, around a rocky outcropping, I encounter a niche in the cliff with a level, sandy floor. I kneel by the bluff and, working against gusts of wind, unroll my blanket awkwardly, crawl into its folds, and wedge my pillow under my head.

The stars wink overhead, serenely still above a driving wind that carries the taste of salt. I hear Reggie telling me to bring my awareness to my breath. She puts a hand on my blanket as if taking the measure of my being. The tension between this intimacy and the elements that immerse us opens a door in my mind. Making love to the sky begins to make sense. I follow her instructions and arch my back as I breathe in, and curl forward as I breathe out. She adjusts my movements until I am rocking gently, easily, and regularly. Then she tells me to touch myself as I please and disappears into the wind.

After a few minutes, I feel a tingling from my tailbone to my crown. Gradually, I learn to pay attention to this sensation, and to amplify it. Waves of subtle energy flow into my lungs, through my spine, and throughout my flesh, which absorbs them like a sponge. The energy waves gradually come into rhythm with the surf. The tingling increases and melds with my heightened awareness. I have never felt so alive, or so awake. I pull the rough edge of my blanket up until I am covered but for my nose and eyes; I rock gently in a cocoon of warmth. Relaxed alertness becomes wonder which becomes amazement. Corporality and carnality join with awareness. I sense that Reggie is supporting me and infer that her energy is catalyzing mine.

This is ecstasy! This is bliss!

I gaze at the stars and welcome them into my eyes, my body,

my being. Andy seems to hover above me, obscuring the sky as he touches me. I allow his hand to act through mine. I rock and breathe and feel his mouth against mine, his hips on mine, his fingers caressing my dewy blossoming labia. I wonder if he can feel me as we move in time with the sea. I fall into a kind of trance. My back opens to the earth, my belly to the stars. I move more quickly. My energy brightens from the center and fills me with light. Andy dissolves into the coverlet of stars, which dissolve into the infinite mystery of creation and destruction. A net of living, tingling stars spreads up my back and joins me to the source of all. I rest in exquisite union with Creation, and tears well up from a place deeper than sorrow. I welcome tranquility and joy. I leave time and awareness.

A hand is steadying my shoulder. Reggie is saying, "Collo, Collo! We're going now."

"Okay." I wrap my arms around my blanket and pillow, jump up and point my feet forward.

I just had a religious experience!

Impossible. Religious experiences are fairy tales.

That was a religious experience. And I had it while masturbating!

Sex and religion are incompatible. Sister Adrian said so! They all say so!

I just felt love with sex. For the first time.

My defenses dissolve. I am exposed, vulnerable, confused. My complacency shatters. I start to sob.

Reggie's arm encircles my shoulders.

"Collo?"

"I'm okay."

"If you're sure," she says dubiously, continuing to hold me. When I calm down, she adds, "Come up when you're ready."

5
Flashback

The night is long, as long as a lifetime of profane gender defilement, a lifetime of victimization and servile accommodation, a lifetime of buried hurts that have been festering in my being. It is a dark night of the soul, the time when demons emerge before they are redeemed. I laugh ghoulishly into my pillow when I realize that Sister Adrian—in making dogma and dependence ridiculous—she pushed me beyond a personified God. Here, my loss of faith is reborn as a growing faith in the sacred heart of life; It is become a pure, undimmed light, able to brighten the darkest beach.

Distorted memories darken that light with phantoms, and sometimes blind my heart entirely, but I am ready for this harrowing. I can turn the horrors of the past into reasons to embrace the whole of my life. The raw material of my transformation comes in like waves, some weak and some strong, some already touched by joy and compassion, some so raw as to give rise to shock and trembling. I am a true Quaker now, as well as a shaker and roller.

I recall—or perhaps dream—that I am in bed with Steven, trying to make love to him. We both laughed at romantics then. We thought that ecstasy and bliss were childish notions and laughed at the idea of sexual connoisseurs. We treated sex as dirty, and felt less and less like having it. When I think of our missed opportunities, my strength fails. I let my tears wash the errors away and try to respect the value of learning things the hard way.

I recall turning towards the wall. I am on the bed naked. The lights are on. The covers are rumpled under Steven's heels. I relive a time I was on top of him, kissing his mouth and gently stroking my swelling labia against his soft penis.

"I'm never going to get hard that way," he whines resentfully. "Why don't you suck me?" Frustrated and humiliated, I blurt, "Because you are five million thrusts behind already."

"What, you always get what you want!"

"It's always over way too fast!"

"It won't be unless you get me up. All you have to do is lie there."

"That's not what I want! You're not paying me, you know."

"You've got a roof over your head, don't you?"

"We should both enjoy it."

"What are you complaining about? You always come."

I slump to the side in cold discouragement. "Forget it. I don't feel like it."

We didn't invent bad sex. Everyone who formed my ideas of sex—from the boys on the playground to the Pope—agreed that sex was naughty and dirty. The nuns taught us that Eve caused the fall and that Mary Magdalene was a whore. Fertility was evil, and all our fault. My eyes sting with self-blame and shame. *How could he and I have botched things so badly?* Steven and I thought we satisfied each other, but we only fucked as if sex eased an unpleasant itch. *We missed every valley.*

What else did we miss? Love. We squandered it. Did we always do that? Yes, says a still small voice. *Yes. We should have found a better way*. People around us made love but we missed it.

I shudder with rage at the realization that generations of girls were reviled for being born, impregnated, and abused. *Why did that happen?* Birth control and feminism had opened new doors, but I missed them. I accepted shame as my burden to bear instead of fighting to love and be loved, body and soul.

I bury my face in my pillow and release waves of old, angry sorrow that rise from the marrow of my legs and exit as hoarse cries. When they pass, I try to open to the grace I'd received on the beach. *Sex can be sacred. It can be worship. It can be a path to the divine. It can open body, mind, and spirit to the sublime.* I reassure myself that even if I never experience it in that way again, I will never forget. It changed my world. I can never be as I was before.

Sometime later, a slow and deep place in my back releases another store of hurt. I am thirteen and watching Carrie, the school slut. She is sitting on the cold asphalt of the playground, smoking a cigarette and eyeing me with petulant defiance. A girl in heavy makeup is combing her hair. I avert my eyes and hurry away, books clutched to my chest in terror. I have been told she is a Bad Girl, and I see her overt sexuality as provocative and dangerous and insulting to good girls like the one I must be.

We are in health class. Sister Adrian is leaning over Carrie's desk. Sister's thin lips are tight above a saggy chin. The purple circles around her eyes look like shiners. "If a boy tries to look up your skirt, or put his hands on your body, you risk damning his soul to hell, too!"

"What if I put my hands down his trousers?"

"That would be a sin to confess to the priest who can bear all of Eve's evils!"

"Should I confess to atom bombs, and the war in Vietnam, and racism?"

"All your sins come from Eve!"

"So now I'm supposed to know the difference between good and evil? Isn't that the original sin?" she retorts smartly.

"Get out of my classroom! There are decent children here!"

Carries goes to the principal's office and never returns. I think a lot about what she said, why she said it, and why she was expelled. I don't want to dwell on it, but can't shut it out. It is the beginning of the end of my faith, but I never speak up for Carrie or others like her, even when I can bear witness to truths reviled by the likes of the unhappy Sister Adrian. I take a shuddering sigh. My heart aches like a fist clenched too long.

As it eases, another wave of stored sorrow is released. This one comes from a place in my heart that once held my cousin Paul. I am doing homework in the living room. He is home from seminary and visiting with Maman in the dining room. He has always been my favorite cousin; he is sweet, good, and kind and has always had a soft spot for me and my girlish troubles. I have no inkling that this is the last time that I will see him.

Right now, he is earnest and angry. He is taking Maman to task. "You must try to be obedient. You must accept the guidance of the Holy Father."

"Of course, Father Paul, I just miss the Latin. It reminded me of French."

Paul's sophomoric tyranny and my mother's apology feel as wrong as a mini-Apocalypse. I go to the dining room to reason with him. "Paul, no one loves the church more than Maman. You know that."

Paul looks intently at the crumbs of fresh brioche on his plate, which she made to please him and to honor his visit. "Many people dedicate their lives to the church, and you know that!"

"You've been in seminary school less than a year. You shouldn't be scolding Maman!"

"I'm going to be a priest. I have to set high standards."

"Paul, why aren't you looking at me? What's got into you?"

"I have to avoid women. Their bodies are inherently evil. They draw men into sin!"

"Paul, I am your cousin! You've known me since I was a baby!"

Paul says nothing, and I leave the room. Later, I hear the door slam. Maman comes in to scold me for failing to show Paul the respect that I owe him as a soon-to-be-priest. When he disappears into the Jesuits, I hear that he is doing good works in Africa, and that his aging mother is struggling alone at home, like mine.

My old embodied hurts continue to arise; I struggle with them. They are almost more than I can bear, and I give thanks that Reggie does not come into our shared bedroom. It is up to me to find strength; it needs to be that way. I find that strength in the recognition that the surface of my life has parted to reveal eternity, giving me a second chance to learn lessons that I was previously unable to receive.

I am not aware of sleeping or of waking; my heart aches for hours. I remain on my side, facing the wall and my errors, trying to release and forgive and transform them so that someday, when I am strong enough, I will be able to extract their meaning and use it to love more broadly and deeply. Right now, they overwhelm me; I have much forgiveness work to do. I must forgive myself, Steven, the Church, and everyone who ever said anything about sex within my earshot, including comedians and priests. *It was the way we were. We mustn't be that way now or in the future. We can learn, become less Rome-like and more Christ-like.*

By the time dawn comes, I am grateful to Reggie for showing me the task ahead, and for offering to help me put my sex life on hold until I learn to sacralize it. I can see that Reggie has been supporting me in this difficult effort by sharing her wholesome state of mind and by guiding me to a way ahead. To calm myself, I relive the day I left Maine for Melbourne, and resumed my stalled journey into the love of life.

Pulling up my hood against the chill Maine air, I watch the steam of my breath lead me towards the lights of my house. Over twenty years ago, I arrived here with my new husband, disappointed that we had put off starting the business that we had planned, and fully expecting to leave when the harvest was in. Since then, life has been a blur of increasing drudgery that I construe as good-natured service. My prayer group regards my acceptance as exemplary; I can hardly bear to think about it.

The usual litany of frustrated problem-solving begins in my mind. I don't realize that it is trying to tell me something. I think of my repeated efforts to begin raising free-range eggs and organic chicken, each of which they barred and ridiculed. I think of my summer job down the coast at Cynthia's bike shop, the job that is keeping the farm afloat and thereby enabling our misery, and then it happens: true acceptance. I accept that as long as I live here, I will never be able to do the right thing.

A still, small voice says, *No one can stop me from doing the right thing.*

I realize with a queasy feeling that today is different. I no longer hope to recover my respect for my husband. I am elated that I never had his children. I have come to see that I will never fit into this family and that they will never show the same regard and responsibility to me that I show to them. I feel odd as I fetch Steve and we go to the main house to eat the dinner that I have cooked for the family and our laborers. I set the table and put out the steaming chicken pot pie that Steve's father always requests, and that Steve's mother always describes as not as good as her mother-in-law's used to be.

As I enjoy the crust that I'd made in my mother's style, I see as if through a spotting scope the beauty of this land, which extends all the way to Maine's Acadia National Park and reminds me of the northern border of my native state of Wisconsin. I love the north woods; the birds, especially the wood ducks; the rugged coast; the outdoor life. I no longer love the indoors. Indoor spaces are too cramped to hold the ill will of this familiy's willful failure.

Steve's father is seated at the head of the table like Oliver Wendell Holmes' autocrat, the man whose house is his domain. He and his wife remember when television came in, and they are still entranced by it. The men—Steve, his father, and the two older single men who live in the old bunk house—bring their low-brow TV shows to the table as jokes about the contemptible qualities of women. I am troubled by the lack of thought and kindness in their lives. When they stopped going to church, they filled its place with smutty antipathy. My spiritual life serves as an antidote. That antidote has been sustaining me since my best friend Christie moved away and took the spirit of our prayer group with her.

"Why do I put up with this?" I ask.

Steve's mother, who is sitting next to me at the foot of the ancient dining table, shoots me a keen glance. "Because you know your place."

"Do I?" I ask with a breathy laugh.

"I should hope you had figured it out by now," she reprimands.

"Me too," I smile. I am not angry; I am afraid of what comes next.

After cleaning up and bidding good night to the joyless old men whose brow hairs block their vision and whose pot bellies silently question my cooking, I follow Steve back to the house. I go to my chair in the den, where I curl up and knit happily until I am able to mute the television that is blurting murder and malice at Steve, who is—as usual—fast asleep on the couch. I take three slow deep breaths and begin my contemplation. I hold all of us in the light and relax into silence. Some minutes later, I try something new: I hold myself in the light.

Before I know it, I have sprung up and grabbed a photo of my friend Reggie, whom I met down the coast when her sailboat was stranded by a gale. Coughlin, the stubborn and suspicious old grocer, was refusing to sell her tampons because she had no American cash and was clearly from some foreign place.

I invited her to lunch and then to stay. Her bright energy enlivened the house, and she enchanted us with stories of bush farms and deserts and billabongs. We spoke French, and she shared bits and pieces of all she had learned in her travels. She took an avid interest in my art and my French country cooking, and I embroidered a vision of our setting up a destination restaurant and winery in the Medoc. When I watched her sails disappear into the light mist of an early summer morning, I realized that she had given me a great gift, a vision of endless possibilities and the hope of pursuing my dream of creative fulfillment.

While gazing at my photo of her, I feel a new clarity and a longing so intense that nothing else matters. Without thinking about it, I go into the bedroom, pack a bag, and go out and start the truck. In minutes, I am on my way to the airport in Montreal. Behind me are my wall quilts of faraway landscapes; my hand-woven blankets, rugs and placemats; my dioramas; and a land that I love. With me, lest I forget, is one diorama of a desiccated marriage that features the skeletons of dormant trees. Ahead of me is faith in life beyond this frozen family, and the story of the new life in which I will do the right thing by the One Life.

6

Denton Stables

By Sunday evening, the pot-au-feu of my being—its ever-simmering stock pot of roots and experiences—is extracting the essential nutrients and flavors of sacred sexuality. A new character and personae are rising to the top—a more creative one that draws on the wilder, unformed essence of life. As we mates chatter and shop on the old high street in Blairgowrie, Reggie and I sense the state of my being, feel it thawing and warming under the Australian sun.

Monday brings with it a more practical new beginning. We pack up to go to Denton Stables, the old stud farm where Reggie and her family are starting up an inn with a destination restaurant, signature winery, and revamped equine facility. As she packs, Reggie explains that Andy and I will be establishing a vineyard while she buys local grapes and begins her exploration of the terroir and of the unpredictable Mount Macedon climate, which at some times brings forth extraordinary fruit and at other times none. When we are not working with her on the viticulture or viniculture, we will help with other tasks such as the remodel of the main house and stables and the construction of guest yurts. Andy will make the same pay that he did at his last job as her assistant at a large winery, and I will receive a small stipend and have the opportunity to find a niche and prove my worth. I am blessed, and feel it as a new vitality.

When we have stacked our suitcases and boxes outside the block of flats, Andy pulls up in the truck. Where we are happy, he is in a snit. I feel no attraction to him now, only amusement and relief as he opens the window and complains a blue streak about suppliers. Andy is my height with broader shoulders and fuller thighs and calves. His features are symmetrical, his jaw broad, and his nose square at the tip below hazel eyes. His wide frame and bronzed fair complexion contrast with my narrow face, raven hair, violet eyes, and winter-pale skin. He pauses to hop out of the red rattle-trap truck that Reggie's family has kept going since the Joads fled the dust bowl in Oklahoma. In it, I will feel like a refugee.

We load the truck and are soon bouncing and squeaking north through mind-numbing, throat-choking, sun-scorched stop-and-go traffic that is punctuated by bursts of tension whenever Andy grips the wheel and honks his horn. This, I expected; but soon something that I have never seen happens between Andy and Reggie: They shift into a fast-forward telegraphic discussion. The lingo goes past me and the context is inscrutable, but I am drawn into their synergy as they burn through problems and fire up solutions. Our minds and hearts join; time dilates; body, mind and spirit serve the action plan that is forming and that I am slowly beginning to follow and to grasp. We are relaxed. We see the way ahead. I want to embody this process and use it for doing the right things at the right time. That would do more to set me on the right path than anything I ever learned before.

North of the city, we emerge into fertile, expansive pasture-lands beyond which the Dividing Range rises gently, much like the mountains of Maine. I love the country and feel at home in it, and compare it plant by plant and stone by stone to the clime I left behind. When we turn right up the road to Mount Macedon, we follow a narrow flat-bottomed valley lined by fields of freshly mown hay and graced by flying clouds of varicolored cockatoos. I am entranced by it until Andy brakes the truck abruptly and we turn into the open gate of Denton Stables, the estate of Reggie's eighty-something grandmother.

As the truck tips away from the tall sandstone fence that lines the highway, I feel a stomach-churning twist, and a surge of relief when the truck rights itself with a jolt. Ahead on the left, a golden sandstone great house rises from a flagstone patio. Opposite, a bridle trail descends to a courtyard framed by stone stables. In the distance, a creek meanders over rolling fields dotted by huge cylinders of hay that lay browning in the morning sun. Near the buildings, tall gum trees form islands of delicious shade that shelter the lawns and gardens.

The old stud farm is as impressive in its signs of new life as in its dying splendor. Some roofs and fences have been replaced, as have scattered broken flagstones and neglected garden beds. The tall grass fields defined by lines of poplars and recently repaired fences are heaped with uprooted prickly pears. The wild bush on the perimeter of the estate is lush despite the dry heat and burning sun. Behind us is a sweeping view of Mount Macedon's rounded shoulder. Reggie says that in the distance ahead, beyond a rise, the land falls away from a stony bluff with panoramic views of Port Phillip Bay. It seems only natural that a family would gather to reclaim the rich potential of this land.

"I can't sort those trellises in a day," Andy complains, with a glance and a tip of his head toward three rows of thick-trunked vines to our left that show that this terrain can serve as wine terroir.

"Maybe Grandma will help you," I joke. Andy snorts and removes his hat to wipe the sweat from his brow. It is the first time that I have seen his full head of maple-colored hair, or noticed the birthmark behind his left ear. My stomach takes a small spin; I am still somewhat drawn to Andy, which is bad for both of us. He and I have become too close, too quickly. I take a deep breath and turn my attention to the object of his distress.

"Did your father put in the vines?" I ask Reggie, who is bouncing along between us.

"He made a little wine here, but those vines have been here for yonks," Andy interjects. "The old lady's used them as bait to get Reg to move up here and play nursemaid."

"No one could make Reg do that against her will," I say.

Andy looks at me with a shitty grin that becomes a leer. It is a teenager tease, and I am embarrassed to find that it lands on me. He is hitting on me and teasing me at the same time. When his desire is intense, mine rises and argues with my reason. I make a mental note to start the celibacy practice tonight. Fortunately, Andy too is holding back. From the whispers that follow him like rustling leaves, Reggie gathers that he keeps his distance from women like me because he does not make women friends and because he is respectful of Reggie's mates.

A hundred yards on, Andy turns abruptly into a grassy drive on the left that leads to the back of the house; he skids and weaves around a large wooden addition behind the house's northeast corner. Beyond a low stone wall that bounds a thriving kitchen garden, we approach a weedy lot. Above us, a picture window overlooks the fields and forest to the east. Ahead, a patio wraps around the far side of the house. On it sits a white iron lace table with four chairs. A big green umbrella rises above a low hedge that encircles the patio except where gaps allow access from the front and back.

Andy stops with a screech that flushes a flock of sulfur-crested cockatoos from a nearby red gum and opens the window he had closed against the dust of the drive.

Reggie says, with a casual air that I realize is forced, "Look, Grandma's a tough old thing, hard of hearing and loud as a galah. She's sharp, though, and a Nosey Parker. Don't say anything you don't want repeated. Best let me do the talking. She has her own way, and does things in her own time. She'll have seen—"

Reggie is interrupted by a shriek, "You can't park there!"

"Grandma!"

Reggie's face registers delight. She gets out of the truck and hurries toward the big umbrella, under which an elderly woman has appeared and is standing and glaring at us. Her hair is dyed bright orange, and she wears a hot pink shift that hangs in soft pleats on her slight form. Wizened but unbowed, she carries a cane in her left hand and waves it at Reggie. Reggie hops over the hedge onto the patio and gives the elderly woman a hug.

Grandma tolerates the embrace and then wriggles free to scold, "Move that truck now, Victoria Regina!"

Reggie darts back toward us. "I'll do it."

Andy and I get out and stand in the shade of a gum tree as Reg follows the arbitrary series of instructions by which Grandma gets the truck into the exact place that she has in mind. It dawns on me that to make a go of it here, we must cater to this crotchety character. Andy and I then follow Reggie to the patio, where Grandma has resumed her seat. After taking time to rest her cane against the table at a particular angle, she commands, "Fetch the tea, now!"

Just then, a tall woman rounds the front corner carrying a tea tray. Her gray hair is precisely cut, her makeup carefully applied, and her posture perfect. Her smile is more distant than warm and more gracious than friendly. Her eyes rest benignly on the tray until I draw her attention by stepping back, at which point her gaze becomes steady and piercing. She puts the tray on the table and says briskly but affably, "Here it is, Mum."

"Grandma, Mum, this is my friend Colette from the States," Reggie says, gesturing toward me.

Grandma's soft spot for Reggie doesn't extend to me. Without looking, she says haughtily, "You may call me Mrs. Elizabeth Denton."

"So pleased to meet you," Reg's mum adds in a British-accented voice. As she hands me a cup of tea and gestures to a chair, she examines my face with benign acceptance. "Please call me Anne."

"How do you do," I reply, taking the cup and my seat. "Thank you for letting me stay at your place in St. Kilda."

Reggie continues, "And this is Andy. You'll remember him from the Cup Carnival."

Mrs. Denton scrabbles for the half-moon glasses that dangle from her neck, sets them high on her nose, and tips her head back to peer at him. "I suppose you're after Reggie's money."

"Grandma, Andy's my top assistant. He's the best in the region, and I can't do without him."

"Hmph. Will he be moving up here with you?"

"Yes."

"Are these two married?"

"Not to each other."

"It's beginning to feel like it," I mutter.

Andy, who is standing behind my right shoulder, mutters,

"Too right." Then he says to Reggie, "I'll have a go at the vines, then, shall I?"

Reggie nods. I see that she is like her mother and grandmother in her confident self-containment, but different in being relaxed and alert, so alert that I always look to see what she is seeing and join my attention to hers. Reggie takes her seat and chooses a scone as the truck starts up and skids away. She commands the mood, but the others are used to this and take no notice, even when her state of being shifts and they align themselves with it.

For the next few minutes, as we sip tea and nibble crumbly scones, I enjoy the delights of the austral landscape and the local architectural style. Given the Devonshire tea, fine china, home-made jam, and clotted cream, I feel like an extra in an Australian production of an English classic novel.

"Where's her husband, then?" Mrs. Denton asks Reggie as she peers at me.

"I'm divorced."

"What's that?"

"She's divorced, Grandma."

"I hope you got your half."

"He didn't have anything to take half of," I laugh.

"A layabout! Why did you marry him in the first place? Was he from good stock?"

"On his mother's side, he could trace his ancestry back to the Mayflower, and to England before that."

"Ah." Mrs. Denton nods and draws herself up. "Our family came over with the First Fleet." After a pause she raises her eyebrows and asks severely, "Why did you divorce him, then?"

"He insisted on living with his mother."

"A layabout with no backbone!" she snorts, adding confidentially, "We've a few black sheep ourselves. Anne married a Levantine, and now his younger son spends his inheritance playing in the sand! At least my Reggie has the Denton character."

"Don't forget Gyorgos," Reggie says. "His new restaurant serves gorgeous food. And beautiful wines, of course. And is more successful than Dad's best. "

Mrs. Denton waves her hand jerkily. "A grown man who cooks all day, and attends an Orthodox church! If he must go to services, he could at least go to Anglican ones! And you, Victoria Regina, it's high time you got yourself a bloke and had a good time while you can!"

Reggie opens her mouth to turn the conversation, but Grandma whacks her shin with the cane.

"After your grandfather had that heart attack, I was glad that we'd made good use of our time in bed. We did it every day. When we couldn't do it any more, he'd watch me with the gardener. For a while he peeped through a hole in the wall, but he got lonely, so he took to sitting in the corner chair."

I glance at Anne, who is looking at Reggie, who is apparently new to this story. I am hoping that Grandma will tire of sharing her strange wisdom, but her story races back through time like a wild brumby galloping past Catholic-Protty conflicts, post-war immigration, the lost generation, the buying of land with dirty money, the deaths surrounding the desecration of song lines, the cannibalism that enabled convicts to reach the bush after escaping prison, and the family myth that their forebears had been transported for stealing bread to assuage hunger rather than for murder. Her rough-edged history and its subtext cut through my romantic notions of my own ancestry, which my parents and teachers edited with silences and elisions, leaving out sources of unspoken guilt and shame, only in old age grappling with past truths written out of official stories.

"You shouldn't miss your chance to breed, Victoria. Why don't you have some fun with that bloke you brought with you? He looks like a stud who'd do you right." Mrs. Denton peers about. "Where is he?"

"He's looking after the vines, Grandma."

"Bring him with you when you move in. And come soon, before I go."

"You look tired, Grandma. Do you want to go in?"

Grandma's shoulders slump; she looks like an empty seed pod that might blow away in a breeze. She sips her tea and puckers in protest, then grabs her cane and rises with difficulty. Reggie rises and offers an arm without the pity or condescension that so many show to frail elders. The two women promenade slowly around the corner, disappearing from sight just as the sun's rays reach over the red gum and touch the stone with golden light.

Anne says, "You're welcome to stay in the flat whenever I'm away. You'd be doing me a service. I don't like to leave it empty."

"Thank you. That's more than kind."

"It's hard being on your own," Anne says with a note of regret. "I know how it is to lose your life partner."

"I'm sorry for your loss." After what I hope is the right interval of silence, I ask nosily, "What does Grandma want from Reggie?"

Anne smiles, revealing a gap between her front teeth. "She wants Reggie and Gyorgos, and Yanni and cousin Geoff, to found an inn that will draw people from Melbourne and overseas. She sees Reggie's wines as the best advertisement, and the inn as a way to fund the stables so that she can take the Melbourne Cup again before she dies."

"And what do you think of her idea?"

"I spend quite a lot of time here, but the estate is hers, and she should do as she sees fit."

"It's a very ambitious plan for someone of her years."

"She has accomplished grandchildren who could carry it out. Geoff is good with horses, Gyorgos has his father's abilities as a restaurateur, and Reggie can make fine wines anywhere."

"What will happen if they don't carry out the plan?"

Anne sighs. "I fear that we will lose the property."

She turns the conversation to lighter topics. She asks if I have visited the National Gallery and recommends an exhibit. When I confess that I have never visited Melbourne on my own, she suggests I explore its gardens and culture.

When a willie wagtail sings in a nearby gum, Anne takes a small pair of binoculars from her purse and lets me watch his tail move from side to side as he lands on a branch. She tells me of the childhood days when she got to know the plants and birds in this place, rode ponies in local holiday races, and participated in the work of the farm. When she asks after my welfare, I tell her of my blue-collar family, my studies, and my marriage and early hopes. When I tell her how things went sour, she frowns and yet waits for me to go on. We are searching for common ground.

I tell her of my Irish and French Catholic roots and of the romantic love that brought my parents together over the objections of their families. My mother, on a rare journey from her Rhode Island mill town, had gone to visit relatives in Chicago, where she saw my father play the fiddle and sing. He entranced her. When he saw her, he responded in kind. When their families objected to their union, they eloped. Poverty forced my father to give up music and to move to Peoria to seek work as a machinist. Both reconciled with their families, but it was too late for my father to recover his vocation, or for us to relocate to an Irish or French community.

When Anne hears this story of a family punishing love with poverty, her expression softens and she recounts her elopement with Reggie's father. Their story was much like my parents'. They moved to the rough neighborhood of Brunswick, where he started a restaurant that became a chain of restaurants. Grandma shunned them until the children were born. As Anne talks, invisible threads of shared experience weave us together. I notice that her dignity and interest in the arts are like Maman's, and that her long skirt, sweet cardigan, and wide-brimmed straw hat reflect an elegant restraint that has left the dark convict past far behind. I wonder if Reggie and I recognized these as central patterns in each other when we first met. I feel accepted, known, and sheltered.

Finally, Anne says, "Let's go in and see if we can find Victoria, shall we?"

Anne scoops up the tea tray and nods toward the linens. I gather them and follow her around the corner of the house, catching her up as she enters the front foyer, which looks disconcertingly like the lobby of my old junior high school. To the right and left—that is to the north and south—wide wooden staircases rise to the balconies that front the upper floors. On the ground floor wall opposite the entry, two sets of French doors open into a formal dining room hung with dingy portraits on the left, and a high ceiling, dark-paneled old ballroom with heavy wood trim on the right. The décor is Victorian with orange and green accents that suggest a mid-century touch-up. The brilliant morning sun halos the open grand piano.

"What grand rooms!"

Anne turns left into a hall that leads into the kitchen addition, which holds an old coal stove and other appliances that are older still. She says absently, "Just leave the linens on the table and go back to the parlor."

I put the linens on a huge butcher-block table in the center of the room and follow the sounds of muted voices back to the long and spacious ballroom now furnished as a library, music room, and lounge room where Grandma is standing with her back to a marble mantle on the left. Her cane is planted on a hearthstone. Reggie sits on an ornate settee facing the hearth, and Grandma seems to be in the middle of a heated interrogation. "Well, then, what kind of tomfoolery are you planning next?"

"Why, Grandma? Have you already scheduled a séance?" asks Reggie.

Grandma Denton lets out an "uh-uh-uh" that seems like outrage but turns out to be a laugh that precipitates a racking cough. Reggie rises and assists her into an armchair, moving easily and lovingly with no hint of force. I take a seat on an old slip-covered armchair beside the settee; its cushion is full of lumps that feel like horsehair.

As Grandma takes the armchair opposite, Reggie explains, "Great-grandma was very attached to her husband. When he died, she had someone come in to do a séance so that she could talk to him. Grandma didn't think much of all that thumping from beyond the grave."

"That fraud was having her on. He'd have had all her money if Uncle Reginald hadn't put a stop to it!"

When Grandma settles, she turns to me and rasps, "Reggie

and I are talking women's business."

"The only business I know is chicken farming."

Reggie smiles. "Grandma's referring to the Aboriginal custom by which women handle some of the family's affairs and men handle others."

"Do you have children?" Grandma interrupts.

"No."

"Do you like women or men or both?"

"Men."

"Then why don't you have a child?"

"I never wanted to have a child with my husband."

"Then why didn't you get someone else?"

"I wouldn't want to raise a fatherless child."

Grandma fixes Reggie with a piercing stare. "I expect both of you to be pregnant by next summer. Can you do it?"

"Is this part of your plan for the stud farm?"

Grandma makes the uh-uh-uh laugh, coughs, and repeats, "Can you do it?"

"I don't know."

"Well, when you get it done, you can come here for your confinement. Mrs. Dean can cook and clean for you. You two can just eat and relax."

I am not sure how to react to Grandma's offer, which is equal parts interference and conniving. I glance at Reggie, who shakes her head slightly. I say nothing.

Grandma continues, "And then we'll put in a new wing and get you a nanny so that you two can give birth to my inn."

Grandma describes her vision for a destination resort that capitalizes on the history of Denton Stables and its role in the racing culture of Victoria. As she speaks of it, she gains energy, leaning forward in her chair and striking her cane against the legs of the furniture for emphasis. She has already acquired several stallions and mares for Geoffrey to breed. Thanks to her knowledge of local bloodlines, she acquired all but one cheaply. That one is the one she intends to race. When she has imparted this, she slumps and says, "Take me up now, Victoria."

I say, "Thank you for the tea. Nice to meet you."

As she leaves, Grandma whacks my shin with her cane, which keeps me quiet and seated while Reggie promenades her slowly out of the room. Then I go back to the kitchen to say goodbye to Anne. She is sitting in a corner furnished with an easy chair with lace-covered arms and headrest. On her left is a side table holding a mug, a lamp, a stack of magazines, and a knitting basket. At her feet is an ottoman. The chair and table sit on a patterned Afghan rug. She has created a small sitting room, a private refuge in the heart of the kitchen that seems a secret pleasure.

"Thank you again. It was lovely meeting you."

"I'm glad you're staying to help Victoria and Andy. My daughter has a lot of friends, but she doesn't see them very often now that she works so much."

"We should change and help Andy with the move to the East stable, Collo," Reggie interrupts. She is standing in the doorway, watching us. "See you, Mum."

Reggie rushes away. I scurry after, saying, "Your Grandma is quite a character. I wouldn't want to cross her. The way she talks about your dad!"

"It's hard to imagine, but Mum's marriage to a Greek was a big scandal back then. Grandma sooked for yonks. But she gave it up when Gyorgos was born, and by the time I was born, our family spent all the holidays up here. Dad and Grandma understood each other. He didn't think much of women, except for Mum and me, but he had a grudging respect for Grandma. She ran this place when Mum was growing up."

"What about your grandfather?"

"He was a free spirit, good with the horses and racing, but not with hiring or firing. He left the business side and the hard decisions to her."

As we make our way down to the stable yard, we see that Andy has parked the truck and is unloading the yurt kits onto the field beyond. I ask Reggie, "You okay?"

"Grandma's driving me mad. I've told her I don't want children, but you see how she is."

"Did she decide that you wanted to help with the inn?"

"Yes and no. Look, don't mention this to Andy yet, but I've got a plan to buy the Greene place in the Yarra Valley. The Greenes are going to retire soon, and they've all but signed the contract. They've got great terroir, and space for more vines; I could sell gorgeous grapes to wineries like Yarra Spur. But I can't bear to tell Grandma. She might—she might give up on life."

"If she insists on controlling every little thing, it'll fail anyway."

"We've a good chance if we give it a go. We grew up with family businesses. We know how to work together."

"What's stopping you, then?"

"The terroir, mainly. I like the taste you can get with the local grapes in a good year, and I'd like to make them into fine wines, but the climate's variable. We'd have to buy grapes, possibly every year. Denton's right for a hobby winery, but not for a qualified oenologist with special expertise in viticulture, like me, or for one of the best managers in the business, like Andy. It's Gyorgos who's driving the project. He's great at start-up, and his menu will draw people from the city. And Yanni can create a weekend sports program. He likes surfing best, but he's always liked racing."

"You're all so different! My family rewarded conformity. In yours, each of you seems to express your own spirit."

"Yanni talks about expressing himself, but I reckon he just wants his way, like me in my wilder days. The solo sailing saved me. It kept me sane and focused and made me strong. Maybe that's why I expect so much of you and Andy."

"I wanted to bring up the subject of Andy," I say shyly.

"I can see you're still attracted to him."

"I like him—in the wrong way. So I'd like to learn the celibacy practice."

"Good. Let's start in the morning."

7

Family Gathering

In the late afternoon of the last Friday in February, as the stable hands who have been helping Andy and me set up the last of the three guest yurts prepare to leave for the day, Reggie comes bounding down the trail from the stable blocks. She has been visiting neighboring vineyards in search of grapes to buy at harvest time.

"Find any sources?" I ask.

"Yes, a couple of good ones. How are you going, Collo?"

"It's amazing how much strength and stamina you can lose in a couple of months! I'm ready to call it quits."

"Couldn't be the heat, could it?" Andy teases with a wink. His teasing has become harmless; my resistance to it has become complete.

"I hope we left enough water for the horses," I say. "We've had gallons."

"Grandma's arranged a dinner meeting. We'll all have to shower and dress by six."

"Is there a problem?" Andy asks warily.

"Probably, but I don't think it's us."

When Reg and I have cleaned up, we go to the bedroom on the third floor of the big house to do our best to dress for the occasion. Reg picks out dresses that Grandma will like, and we tart ourselves up like city girls.

"Hoy, Reggie!" a woman's voice calls from the bottom of the stairway.

Reggie replies, "We're up top, Melanie. Come up, if you like."

I hear heavy steps on the stair and turn to see a bright and beautiful young woman with long sun-bleached hair laboring upward. Her head bobs above the top step, and then her pregnant belly follows. She appears to be eight months along.

"Oh! Hullo, there," she says when she sees me.

"This is Colette Connolly, my friend from the States. She's working with Andy and me on the wines and reno. Colette, this is my sister-in-law, Melanie."

"We were going to work here, too, before we moved to Lorne."

"Lorne?"

"It's near Bell's Beach, the big surfing beach on the Great Ocean Road."

"You're married to Yanni?"

Melanie smiles brightly, nods, and asks eagerly, "Are you from Chicago?"

"I've been living in Maine, but I grew up in Illinois."

"I thought I heard it in your accent. All those nasal 'uh' sounds."

"You have a good ear. Have you spent time in the States?"

"I did a year of university in Chicago."

I feel as if we are friends already. "Oh, my goodness! I went to University of Wisconsin!"

Reggie looks on with amusement as Melanie and I proceed to exchange the histories of our lives. Her partner is Reggie's younger brother Yanni, a passionate surfer dedicated to perfecting his skills and winning tournaments. Melanie says that she believes her love will steady and redeem him, turning him into the father he is poised to become.

Where Reggie is true, kind, and constant, Melanie is warm, light, and responsive. As we share our favorite experiences of Melbourne, we approach the verge of effervescence.

Once we are dressed, Melanie puts her hand under my elbow and leads me down the stairs and into the brightly-lit ballroom. She demurs as the rest of us drink sherry and wait for Grandma, who likes to arrive last and to lead a ready procession into the dining room. I glance at the décor and the guests, and do a double take; I think I am seeing a second Reggie, but then realize that I am looking at Yanni. He is approaching with their older brother Gyorgos. As they near us, I see that Yanni has a thicker jaw than Reggie, as well as lighter and sun-tipped hair.

Grandma enters, and we follow her from the ballroom into the dining room via the east doors that join the two. Grandma's style is old fashioned but flattering. She is wearing a long-sleeved, high-necked dress and her hair is pinned up in a chignon. She takes a seat at the head of the table, from which she has a commanding view of the east pasture and the forest beyond. Reg sits on her left, and Gyorgos; Ruth and Andy sit beside Reggie. Gyorgos is shorter and darker than Reggie, with close-set, dark brown eyes and an imperious expression. His much younger wife Ruth has a petite narrow face framed by dark hair and straight brows. When she regards her husband, she glows with a look of sweet adoration. Anne sits on Grandma's right; next to her sits Yanni, and then Melanie, Geoffrey, and me. I realize with a jolt that I can feel Yanni's sexual magnetism all the way at the end of the long table, and that this energy makes him appear to be drop-dead gorgeous.

Reggie opens a bottle of wine, pours an ounce into her glass, then passes the bottle to Gyorgos as she introduces me formally to the family.

Gyorgos fixes me with a piercing stare and asks, "Where did Reggie find you?"

"On the coast of Maine, when she was sailing around the globe."

"Oh, that trip!" Melanie exclaims. "She nearly went down that time, didn't she? Got caught out in a storm on Bass Strait. It was in all the papers."

"Don't remind me. I was a national laughingstock," Reggie says.

"Reggie said it taught her patience," Ruth adds, "but it taught us panic."

"Collo here rescued me from a different storm," Reggie says.

"Do you sail?" Yanni asks.

"No! What Reggie means is she stayed at our farm for a few weeks while she waited for good weather. Gave her a chance to practice her French."

"Well then, thank you for rescuing my sister, and welcome to the family!" Gyorgos declares. He raises his glass to me. The rest quickly pour out wine and raise their glasses to toast me; I realize that they are accepting me because Gyorgos has signaled his approval. I wonder if they are bowing to his authority, or merely pretending that he is in charge.

After the toast, Reggie says, "Yan, why don't you tell us of your plans for the baby."

Yanni starts warily, but soon warms to his story of surfing when the waves are good and loafing when they are not. He plans to ride the waves to championships around the world while

Melanie stays home to work and care for the child, dipping into his inheritance as needed. His train of thought soon wanders into tales of drinking with his mates and teaching his son to surf. His words reveal an interior that is wild, careless, and childish. When others ask brief questions, it becomes clear that he has never held a job or stayed with a woman for more than six months, and that he is paying little or no attention to the family venture.

I watch Gyorgos watching Yanni. Gyorgos seems to be wound up to spring when the time is right; he waves his broad hands and shifts his heavy carpet of black hair. I remember now that Gyorgos became the patriarch of the family when their father died. As Gyorgos became steadier and more ambitious, Yanni became wilder.

Gyorgos gestures toward Yanni and declaims, "You make me ashamed to be a Pappas!"

Shock registers on all faces, especially Yanni's. I infer from this that both brothers take pride in the name of Pappas, and that Yanni's pride depends on his older brother's approval. Yanni gives Reggie a resentful look, as if to say that she has Gyorgos' good opinion, but shouldn't. Then he looks darkly at me. I look at Melanie, whose glow of love now seems to be born of hormones that have blunted her reason.

I notice that Ruth is wearing a necklace that displays a large gold cross in the Greek Orthodox style; I remember that she converted when they married, and became a typical religious neophyte anxious to conform to strict standards. She is unlikely to countenance Reggie's practices—or mine—or to be in sympathy with Yanni. I feel tension rise around the table, and wonder if Yanni will try to take advantage of family fracture lines.

Melanie says sweetly, "You're proud of your Greek and

convict roots, Gyorgos. Yanni is too, and our baby boy will be. I'm with Yan one hundred percent, and so are his friends. Most of them have kids and can't wait for Yan to have one, too. We know what we're doing, don't we, Yan?"

Yanni is transformed. Melanie loves him. When he is holding her hand, he loves her, too, and seems to merit his beauty and his family. There is hope when he is thinking of her; he holds steady as his siblings admonish him to take responsibility for his life. When they say that they value Melanie and the baby, and hope that Yanni will deserve them rather than lose them, he nods soberly. Gyorgos ends by saying that he expects Yanni to be a model for his children as their father was for them, and as Gyorgos is for his. Yanni, still holding tightly to Melanie's hand, vows to be so. The moment is pregnant with the possibility that Yanni may use his partnership and fatherhood to embrace the fullness of his manhood.

After the dinner that Gyorgos did not prepare and that the family barely tastes, we return to the parlor, where Andy and I move to one side and discuss the placement of the vine trellises while the others catch up on family business. After a few minutes, Grandma commands Reggie to escort her up to her room, and the family flocks quietly out into the vestibule and then into the kitchen.

Andy and I, puzzled, follow and watch as, like Darwin's finches, each member of the family finds a niche. Gyorgos goes to the old woodstove that was converted to gas and that dominates the north wall. There he begins a noisy, rapid juggling act that works in the pots and pans suspended above the stove, a row of grocery bags sitting on the big butcher block table, and a set of knives that he has unrolled near a convenient chopping area that he has wiped down. Ruth has cornered Melanie in the pantry and is cross-examining her about vitamins and nutrition. Yanni has taken two of the skateboards stacked by the door that leads to the kitchen garden and gone out to find Gyorgos' young boys and their babysitter.

Anne is sitting in the easy chair in her corner refuge, knitting. Geoffrey enters with a dining chair that he places close to her calm and nurturing presence. He has switched from wine to scotch, and is on his fourth drink. He holds his liquor like a regular and glances at the others warily. I did not notice at first that he was gay—my gay-dar does not work down under—but it may explain why he takes pains to keep his distance and only tolerate me as Reggie's friend.

I whisper to Andy, "How do we find our place in this family nest?"

"Buckley's chance." He retrieves a newspaper from Anne's basket of pulps and glossies, sits on one of the stools on the near side of the table, and proceeds to read.

I stand for a moment, enjoying the warmth of a loving, engaged family gathered around its hearth, and then notice that Gyorgos is stacking dirty pans and utensils in the triple sink by the door that leads out to the kitchen garden. I take it as my cue: I go to fill the sink with soapy water and, elbow deep in suds, wash and stack the dishes on a towel beside the sink.

I let my mind wander, and it follows familiar associations into the distant reaches of my childhood. I am sitting in my highchair in the corner of the kitchen watching Maman mix a bowl of elastic dough. Melissa claims that I cannot possibly recall such an early event, which may be true or may reflect the questioning of everything that came with her illness. In this memory, I bang on the shiny aluminum tray to catch Maman's attention so that she will take away the hard, shiny boiled egg glistening in the white ceramic cup. I am not hungry, and do not want it. I tell her, but she does not understand my speech, or does not take my point. She beams at me with the exquisite tenderness at the magical center of her sea of motherly love. I accept that I must speak more clearly, and so push my egg over the edge of the tray onto the floor far below. She is infinitely forgiving, then, and so laughs and comes to clean it up.

I am standing on a chair at the stove. I must be old enough to be trusted by the gas fires. I extend the tip of my tongue to lick away a soft dot of flour on my wrist. I do not remember the taste on my tongue, but I recall the feel of stirring Maman's thickening Béarnaise sauce, and of gripping the smooth handle of her wooden spoon. I extend my arm farther than ever before to try and reach a dented can of sugar and cinnamon. I can still feel the exertion of kneading a first gooey dough; the pressure exerted in rolling out a long crust in Maine; the ridge of a curl of carrot cut by my brother's wife in New Orleans; the flipping of an omelet in Anne's St. Kilda kitchen. It is the movements of the culinary arts that reside in me, like a repertory of dance moves.

I have a vision of myself wearing a chef's hat and holding a knife at the ready, and I realize that I have found my vocation. I long for the sweet taste of caramelized onions, the gut-filling satisfaction of a fatty steak, the hearth fire deep below the navel that fuels vitality and impels me to create a cuisine that in turn creates a community like this. My vocation of artist expands to encompass the kinesthetic pleasures of dicing, of lifting the heavy lid of a saucepan, of scraping a frying pan. These awaken my palate; I taste savory oregano, tangy wine vinegar, and musky portobello. My vocation is joining the engines of vitality to an art that began many millennia before the dawn of cultivation, and that will linger as long as humanity. I will engage my fine art skills in nurturing this whole-body art that flows from the sun through soil and seeds to the palate and stomach.

A light goes on outside. Yanni and the three boys—Gyorgos' sons Taki and Barry and their sitter Ethan—have set out plywood and ramps, and Yanni is teaching them simple maneuvers. Looking up now and then as I dry some dishes and wash more, I see Ethan and then Taki do ollies—a maneuver in which they jump up, flip the board, and land on it again. Yanni is a good teacher.

I notice that I am unexpectedly heartened, and think that it's the slippery feel of the dishes, or the squeak of a damp towel on crockery. Then I look around and see that Reggie has rejoined us in the kitchen and is holding us in loving equanimity. I do what I can to add my energy to hers.

It seems only minutes later that Gyorgos is serving us an improvised dinner of spinach feta soufflé, rare roasted eye fillets on a bed of mango-accented skordalia, a wilted salad with crispy onions, and baklava from one of his restaurants. The aromas are enticing. When we have taken seats on stools around the butcher-block table, I tentatively taste each dish and am enchanted by his creativity.

"Oh my God!" I exclaim. "Your palate is extraordinary, Gyorgos. How could your restaurant *not* succeed?"

Gyorgos looks at Reggie who looks at Yanni. They say in unison, "Grandma."

Anne says placidly, "The old dear still feels responsible for everything, but has no idea how things have changed."

Gyorgos throws his hand up and says, "She's impossible! None of the local caterers will work with her."

Ruth adds quietly, "She always wants something for nothing."

Gyorgos ignores her and continues. "She insists on serving the worst food! She's long since lost her taste and smell—but still pretends she hasn't!"

Ruth says, "If only she would give Gyorgos a free hand—" she stops abruptly as Gyorgos shoots her a glance of warning. Ruth turns her attention to her food and says "—she could eat as well as this at every meal." She smiles at me and finishes her skordalia.

Anne says diplomatically, with a knowing look at Gyorgos, "Grandma is losing her vitality as well. I doubt you'll be seeing her in the kitchen."

"She still counts every coin, though, doesn't she?" Yanni snorts.

"She's paying for everything. She only wants to know her money isn't wasted," Reggie says kindly.

I feel a surge of dark energy and realize that I am sitting equidistant from Reggie and Yanni, who are facing each other across the table. Her loving compassion has intensified, which seems to only feed his contained rage. I recall my childhood anxieties about purgatory, which I imagined to be at the border of heaven and hell. Unsettled, I look at the others. They do not seem to notice the love-hate bond between Reg and Yanni. I am impressed by Andy's detachment; I realize that he has a high tolerance for conflict and is well able to keep his composure.

Anne looks at me and clears her throat. Yanni looks at his plate, and his state shifts abruptly into that of obedient child. The others stops eating and look at her expectantly.

"Geoffrey's been punting again. His gambling addiction has

gone out of control. He and I have talked about it and set some limits to protect the Stables and the inn. I want all of you to help by refusing to stake him or to allow any of our associates to do so, and to feel free to use all but the racing horses for riding."

Yanni frowns and objects, "He's always saying that all the horses are for racing only!"

"The rides will exercise all of the horses that will not race."

Everyone looks at Geoffrey, who feigns interest in a piece of lint on his lapel.

"Is that what you want?" Melanie asks him kindly.

Geoffrey nods and affects boredom.

Anne turns to Yanni. "Gyorgos is preparing the meals and making most of the arrangements for the inn. Victoria and her mates are doing the same for the viticulture and viniculture. It's time you organized the sport programs. What do you have in mind?"

I can feel fear rise in Yanni as he replies, unsteadily, "I could set up a skate park and coach skaters and lead horse rides if we can use the horses." His voice falls as he looks at his mother; his lack of confidence is obvious.

"He's a good teacher," I say.

"How do you know?" Taki asks curiously.

"I saw him teach you to do an ollie."

"Skaters aren't known as big spenders," Ruth says.

"Their parents may be," Melanie says.

"Good," says Anne. "I'd like you to show me your progress next Wednesday. You'd best stay here and work on it until then."

Yanni grunts displeasure but doesn't object.

"You and Melanie can stay in the finished unit in the South Stables."

The dinner conversation resumes slowly. Anne finishes eating last. She and Ruth and I clear the table and wash the dishes while Yanni and Melanie go to the South Stables, Gyorgos and Reg return to the parlor, and Geoff goes to look in on Grandma, who has the habit of going to sleep with her candles lit. Andy returns to his paper. When Anne and Ruth go up to their rooms, I fetch a sketchpad, pencil, and pastels and return to draw while I drink a refreshing tisane.

Reggie enters, sits with a groan, and kicks off her high heels. "The good news is, Gyorgos is trying his new menus on his old school mates, and he'll be opening on Saturday nights by invitation only. The bad news is we'll be making room for him and his family by moving to the West Stables."

Andy sits up and stares at her askance.

"The ones not fit for man nor beast?"

"We have two days to make the upstairs rooms fit for us, which means we'll have to put off everything else for a bit."

"Where will we stay tonight?"

"The tent at the practice track? Geoff's set it up as an office that he could do without."

"Good thought."

As they talk it through, I bask in the esprit de corps that we are forming and reflect that here, now, we work together smoothly and are each at our best; together we are more than the sum of us. Andy is focused and engaged and wastes no energy in teasing or griping or giving in to impulses that derail his purposes. I am as creative and alive as I have been in years, and free of distracting inner conflict and confusion. Reg is able to realize plans that she cannot effect alone.

"What are you sketching?"

"I have an idea."

"Let's have it," Andy says.

"I've realized that I'm a chef, and that I want to be Gyorgos' apprentice in the kitchen."

Reggie looks surprised. She looks at Andy as if to find out if he expected this, and then says, "You certainly know your way around a kitchen. I love your crêpes and brioches. And you had the same problems with the family in Maine that Gyorgos has with Grandma."

"And Gyorgos will need help if none of the foodies here will work for Grandma," I say.

Andy asks with a sly grin, "But can you make a meat pie? I'll be needing some fair dinkum tucker if I'm good to be doing some hard yakka."

"Actually, yes," I reply. "I can. Fish pie, too."

"What about the art?" Reggie asks.

"My idea is to trade art for training."

"Let's have a look, then."

I set out the sketches. One is of a mural for a yurt, and the other is of a mural for the entry wall between the doors to the living and dining rooms. The yurt mural is a painting of racing horses and gum trees that combines visual references to Grecian urns and racing photos, and which features earth tones that incorporate the colors of the built and natural environments. The one for the entry wall is a primitivist still life of flowers in a vase, two from each of the continents, with hyper-realistic miniatures at the center of each bloom that show scenes characteristic of that continent. One of the European miniatures is an iconic image of the island of Santorini.

"They're gorgeous! And rooted in tradition but global and

dynamic and fresh. Just what we want. But I'm afraid you'll have to let us pay you for the art, and for your work as a chef—if Gyrogos agrees to take you on."

"They'd brighten up this funeral parlor. When's the last time the old lady redecorated?" Andy asks.

"I don't think she did." Reggie's tone turns to concern as she asks me, "How are you going with the family? I saw you clocking Yan and me."

"I feel that you and Andy and I are forming a community that I love more than any family that I've been part of, and I'm hopeful that this project will bring out our best. I feel at home. Fingers crossed for Yanni; I'm not as hopeful about him."

Andy stands, pushes aside his stool, and folds his paper. "I'll leave you two to your hen party."

"Goodnight," I say with a smile.

"Right-o," Reg says contentedly. "Let's work out a strategy for getting you into the kitchen."

"I thought women didn't want that any more," Andy says over his shoulder before disappearing toward the entry.

"This one does," I reply with a smile.

8
Birthday Party

I turn the crank handle of the top wire strainer. Andy nods, and we move down the lyre trellis to the next angled post. This careful turning will enable the rootling vines to grow and develop, and so to shape the future of The Inn at Denton. Andy has put in many posts and wires, and the wind is playing them like an instrument. He is teaching me to tell by pitch as well as by feel when the wires are tight enough to anchor the new rootlings, and yet loose enough to remain resilient in rough weather.

We started at the rise of the weak August sun, as has become our habit, and plan to take breaks: me to help our chef create new recipes, Andy to help Yanni complete the hothouse that they are building from scavenged scraps. That north-facing incubator, which stands at the center of the sheep-dotted north pastures, looks like a rubbish heap huddled against the remnants of Denton's first stone dwelling; inside it feels like an Eden, and we are filling it with planters that will serve the restaurant well.

Another motor speeds down the drive toward the house. I ask, "Who is it now?"

"You trying to get out of some fair dinkum yakka?"

"You're as curious as I am, and you know it. Besides, now that we're part of this crazy scheme, it's our duty to know what's going on."

"It's our duty to finish up and go down to the pub."

"Did you know that Grandma knew this many people?"

"She knows everybody in country Victoria, and everyone else who has followed racing since time began."

"A lot of them must want to wish her well on her ninetieth birthday."

"They want a free meal, and they know that this time she can't fire the caterer at the last minute."

I kneel and adjust the bottom strainer; the handle slides into the purpling bruise in my palm. I pause to shift my grip and reflect for a fleeting moment on the creative center of this nascent venture. Andy and I are playing roles at its periphery, often in the fields, at a remove from the vision and the decisions that Reggie and her family are forming. We are actors, not authors, for this intergenerational saga. We support them and cheer them on but have little say—and less responsibility.

"I can't wait to try the new dishes Gyorgos developed for this dinner," I say.

"I thought you were making an aspic."

"That's for the lunch buffet. Dinner will be an exclusive preview of his new Asian–Greek fusion cuisine. It's white tie and everything."

"I'll give that a miss, then."

"You can't leave me alone with that family! I'll never recover. And then you'll have to plant the new rootlings all by yourself."

"Might as well, with all the time you've been spending in that kitchen. Do you fancy Gyorgos?"

"I fancy his talent, and his skills."

Andy and I reach the end of the row and move on to the next. A gust raises fine, sharp grit that stings our skin. I close my eyes to protect them, crank the strainers, and check the tension by feel. We work as one all the way to the north pasture, where I take a break to admire the trellises that raised the new crop of calluses on my hands and that are binding me to Andy as a co-worker.

A flight of pink cockatoos flaps against the wind that is pushing up the Great Dividing Range from the Southern Ocean. They clear the knob of Mount Macedon, then the farm to the north of the road, and then the zither of wires strung between the sheep-dotted north pastures of Denton Stables and the drive along which the guests are coming in for Grandma's ninetieth birthday celebration.

At the end of the next row, I kneel and pause to look up at the cockatoos, who are returning to the mountaintop on a mysterious errand. I lean back and let the wind run up my chest, thinking of my friend Carolyn, who spent a month in Kauai every winter, living wild and learning the hula. She taught me the *hula noho*, in which the dancer kneels and leans back to listen to the voices in the wind.

When Andy raises a dubious eyebrow, I stand and say, "Just listening to the voices of the ancestors."

Andy nods approval of the wire tension, and we move down the row. "Now you sound like my wife."

"Thank you."

"It wasn't a compliment."

"What do they say to her?"

"If they had any sense, they'd say we should leave this place as soon as Reg gets a babysitter for Grandma."

I drop my hands in dismay. "Are you saying this is busywork?"

Andy motions for me to keep cranking. "Reg'll give this toy

to one of the family to manage. They don't need someone like her for this."

"Don't call our baby a toy."

"This isn't our baby. We'd do better."

Andy is right; this trellis is the product of our sweat and our limbs, not our blood or our spirits. His blood is bound to Lisa, his Indonesian refugee wife, and his spirit to his work. I am on fire to master the art of living, and to transmit it to a community of spirit children, perhaps by fulfilling the dream of founding a winery with a restaurant and a retreat center. I like to imagine that our work here is preparing us to do that at some indefinite time in the future.

As we turn at the end of the row and exchange roles so that I am checking the tension, another car passes, and Andy asks, "Who is it now?"

"Melanie. Back from the Queen Victoria market."

"I'm surprised Gyorgos didn't go."

"He's still figuring out the commute and prepping his suppliers to give what he wants to her." I add tentatively, "You seem a bit off today."

Andy takes off his bush hat, runs his hand up over his square features and back over his short-cropped hair, and pulls up his broad shoulders. He presses his lips together, and after an unusual pause, says, "Lisa's pregnant and she's on her way out here to talk about it."

"Congratulations?"

"The timing's terrible. She's living at home with her family now—with parents who speak no English and hate me even though they practically forced her to marry me. We were saving money to buy a place and we need it because she's barely stable when we're alone—she's come at me with a knife more than once—and I reckon she'll be worse here."

Andy has never confided in me this way. I snuff out my shock and do what I can to take his confidence in stride, as if it doesn't change everything. "I'm so sorry to hear that."

"Lisa's had it rough. Grew up in Indonesia. Saw carnage, barely escaped. Still doesn't feel safe. Worries that their enemies will come and kill them. Her father was quite the troublemaker back home." Andy snorts and corrects himself. "Troublemaker! I reckon he was genocidal."

"Where? Against whom?"

"Does it matter?"

"I just ... I don't know how to think about it."

"You can't. You can only love and hope. Bloody mess is what it is."

"A baby can change a life, maybe even be the best thing that could happen after something like that."

Andy sighs tensely.

"Can Reggie give you all a place to live?"

Before Andy can speak, Reggie's voice calls out happily from down the pasture, "Grandma's invited everyone she knows. I reckon we've sparked the old doll."

Andy stands and stretches his arms with showy unconcern. Reggie approaches and puts her hand on the wire we just tightened. She gives us a glowing smile. "Great work on the trellises. Let's go over to the hothouse and organize the tomato planters before we have to dress for lunch."

Andy drops his tools and says with unconvincing disgust, "I'll get that started. Have to leave time to brush up the penguin suit."

As he lopes away toward the north pasture, I ask Reggie,

"Andy owns a suit?"

"He keeps a few for formal and informal business events."

"Is lunch going to be formal?"

"We can wear smart casual at lunch, but with Grandma it's white tie for dinner."

"I don't have any evening wear."

"I'll bring up the green gown for you, and the silk shawl."

"Thanks. It'll be like playing dress up."

"It should be great fun sharing Grandma's pleasure."

I back away down the gentle decline of the north field. "I should go down now and finish the aspic before lunch."

"Aspic? I haven't had an aspic in donkey's years."

"No one has, which is the reason it offers a wonderful opportunity for creativity. I'm experimenting with heightening the flavors and playing with the presentation. Today's effort will be a wiggly amber cake with dill and fennel gel, and a ring of whipped pink peppercorn cream."

"Can't wait."

I feel new, and newly sanguine, when darting through the kitchen door and on to the bathroom beyond to shed my dirty field clothes and prepare to cook. As the old water heater clanks on, I freshen in a lukewarm shower, put on a fashionable outfit, and go to mingle with the finely-dressed guests who are crowded into the living room and foyer. Some examine my mural, which is nearly finished, and others enjoy the collection of Melbourne Cup hats that Melanie found in the attic and hung on the walls on the other sides of the French doors. The hats add color, muffle the foyer's noisy echo, and set off the mural.

Amongst the strangers who are sipping cocktails and sharing gossip about horses, families, and business are Reggie's university friends Louis, Emily, Roger, and Judy. When I press through the crowd to greet them, I see that they are talking with another group that includes Dutchy and Hal, who says immediately, "I love the murals! Can we commission a painting?"

I feel the stress of being asked to do more, and yet am flattered and grateful. "Thanks, but not anytime soon. Right now I'm apprenticed to Gyorgos."

"You're going to be a sous-chef? What a wasste!" Dutchy says in dismay.

"I hope not? Try my aspic and let me know what you think," I laugh.

I bid them good appetite and goodbye, and plunge through the crowd into the kitchen to assemble the aspic that I put in the refrigerator last night. Gyorgos is orchestrating the meal from the butcher-block table, where he is plating dishes for the Scandinavian smörgåsbord he designed for the luncheon buffet; they will serve as a counterpoint to the Greek–Asian fusion cuisine that he will unveil this evening.

Gyorgos is calling out instructions to two assistants he hired from the neighborhood, the young Eva, a mahogany-haired girl with round features and big eyes who is frying small discs of sheep cheese as a topper for onion and lemon canapés, and Bryan, her taller and darker older brother who is frying root vegetables to make colorful chips for roe dip flavored with dill. Though Eva is still in high school, and her brother has only just graduated, they belong to a neighboring family of winemakers and have a sophisticated grasp of the culinary arts.

Gyorgos calls out, "Colette! Sharpen the knives!"

I put on a tall white chef's hat and apron, hurry the aspic out to the shelf atop the display table in the dining room, and return to sharpen the knives on the whetstone with a sweep clink, sweep clink, sweep clink, sweep clink. Then it's cut, cut, cut onions into precise slices, moving fingers steadily back and blade steadily on, and turning the resultant thin slices to cut, cut, cut those into tiny cubes.

Already, sharp and mild aromas and flavors are infusing the kitchen's aromatic breath with a new world of taste. Like the revolution in European cuisine following the increase of the spice trade, Gyorgos' new synthesis joins ingredients, traditions, and skills that arose here and all around the globe, and educates palates in his mix of farm-bred herbs, ovine cheeses, bush tomatoes, and root vegetables.

Like his wine-making sister, Gyorgos holds the keys to mastering one of the arts of sensual intimacy that interpenetrates the infinitely innovative web of life. Until now, I have practiced cooking as a craft rather than an art, and still do not like Gyorgos' imperious and exacting manner, which is unpleasantly intense for Eva and Bryan: they are unaccustomed to city manners and suspect him of being no more than self-important. Where Reggie is open and welcoming, Gyorgos treats us as he treats himself, as laborers rather than as sisters, brothers, partners, or apprentices. Eva and Bryan are even more skeptical of Reggie than of Gyorgos; she takes the Ayurvedic view that taste seeks out flavors that fill subtle bodily lacks in minerals or other nutrients and qualities. They think it strange that she trusts the wisdom of taste by offering a selection of wines at the table and encouraging diners to take what appeals. To me, her wines seem to flow like streams through the landscape of Gyorgos' Greek-influenced cuisine, tumbling over and under spices and herbs, cutting through textures and reshaping flavors.

I am still elated by my new vocation. Every meal we make is the best I've ever eaten, every nuance of flavor and texture pregnant with delight and surprise. Eating is never dutiful or compulsive; each course is worthy of note, and every meal creates a unique afterglow. As I cut carrot flowers to add color to the presentation of the buffet, I hear Gyorgos call from the dining room, "Colette! Come here now!"

I wink at Eva and hurry to the linen-clad buffet table, where Gyorgos is standing and staring at the top tier with an expression that suggests that my aspic platter is an insult to cuisine. Indeed, in its elevated position, its fluffy ring of dill garnish looks like a pile of weeds. Gyorgos pulls off the dill and holds it out to me like a dirty diaper. "The gelatin is firm. The eggs and fish made a good pattern. Frame it, don't feather it."

I laugh. "It does look like one of your mom's old Cup Day hats."

"Reconceive!" Gyorgos commands, raising both hands expansively.

I take the plate to the kitchen and ring it with wilted chard, quartered hardboiled eggs, and carrot flowers. Then I return it to the table and assist Eva and Bryan as they bring out string beans with almonds, rye bread, cheese blocks, and other dishes to complete the smörgås, including warm ham and iced salmon. When Gyorgos has inspected the table and altered it to suit his aesthetics, he calls the guests to lunch.

For the next two hours, Gyorgos hosts as the three of us serve. We take advantage of our easy informality with the family party to discover shortcomings, like the need for more fresh dinner plates. When the ritual is finished and nearly all the diners have vacated their seats, we return to the kitchen, remove our aprons and hats, and hang them on the newly painted wall beside the copper pots. We organize a lunch plate of cheese and apples and toast and share it at the butcher-block table.

Soon, members of the family enter one by one, each ostensibly looking for a snack, but in fact hoping to hear Gyorgos' thoughts about serving a meal to the public in this place. Soon, Melanie and Niko, Ruth and her children, and Anne all join us at the table, while cousins straggle in and idle in the sitting area and along the inner walls.

A girl of seven or eight pulls on Anne's skirt. "Auntie, I'm hungry."

Just then, Reggie enters. I hurry over to Anne, give the girl my plate of cheese and fruit, and say, "Reggie, can I have a word?"

Reggie's face registers surprise. "If you like."

"Come this way." I lead her into the hall, and then into the old bathroom.

"What's the matter?"

"I want to talk with you about Gyorgos' creative engagement with the culinary arts."

Reggie gives me an odd look.

"He's really inspiring!" I start to gush, aware that I am sounding like a groupie, but unable to stop. "His palate is so discerning, and his imagination is daring without being outlandish, and he can realize his creative ideas with clarity and simplicity. He's incisive—almost Zen—in the way he focuses on sources and keeps the preparation and presentation simple. His style is as elegant as yours, and Maman's. It's almost French."

"I reckon you'd find finesse in any culinary tradition," Reggie says with an amused smile.

"Including new ones that integrate East and West, like your spirituality does. Which is why I'd like your blessing to do a different mural on the third yurt—a food and wine one."

"Absolutely. Lovely idea. I'll take care of your work in the hothouse, free you up to focus on painting and cuisine."

"Thanks! That'll help me focus."

Soon, Gyorgos orders everyone else out of the kitchen and inspires his team with his vision of renewing Greek cuisine by giving it an Asian twist. The menu will begin with an appetizer of wonton dough stuffed with spinach and feta, brushed with olive oil, baked and presented on a plate drizzled with avgolemono sauce. The first course will consist of steamed egg custards with lamb broth, ground lamb, ginko nuts, and mint. The second will include roasted lemon chicken on a bed of mashed skordalia with a side of shiitake souvlaki, and another side of long beans with Greek herbs. The dessert will be the lychee baklava we made yesterday. It is a bold effort designed for food lovers whose lives have extended beyond old borders. The room is filled with the excitement we feel on participating in its debut.

"Did you consider a bed of rice with a side of skordalia and long bean fritters with cilantro pesto?" I ask. "That brings in the key flavors as well as the deep-fried course expected in a kaiseki meal."

Gyorgos stops. His mouth is open, and his right hand holds a cleaver that is pointing toward the hammered copper kettles hanging above our heads. Eva and Bryan look down. I wince in expectation of an outburst. But Gyorgos makes a small puffing noise and says, "Not bad. Next time."

We go into high gear, but within the hour, the orderly kitchen has devolved into uncharacteristic chaos. We have not yet finished the broths or sauces; food debris is scattered on the floor; and dirty dishes are stacked in the sink. Gyorgos has shifted from his search for perfection to looking for shortcuts that won't spoil the meal. As his hands fly above the stove and we execute his precise commands, the intensity of our preparation becomes pleasurable, and we reach a new level of coordination working side-by-side and in sequence toward the same moment in time.

Abruptly, Gyorgos' ephemeral creations are almost ready for family-style service. Eva and Bryan begin cleaning up the kitchen, and Gyorgos and I go to put on formal dress. After a hasty shower, I wipe the steamy mirror and put on makeup and the dress and shawl that Reggie left hanging on the back of the door. When I step out into the dark and deserted foyer, she is waiting in an ankle-length, deep purple velour and silk gown that brings out her beauty.

"You look amazing."

"I reckon Grandma was right to have us dress. It makes for a break, sets the right tone for a destination restaurant."

"Where do we go?"

"We're gathering in what you call the living room."

Reggie makes a dramatic entrance by opening the French doors with one sweeping motion that draws the attention of the entire extended family, who are gathered around the hearth where Grandma is standing and leaning on her cane. She is wearing a sexy dress from the 1930's that she has covered with a feather stole, her hair drawn up in a French twist. When she sees Reggie, she bangs her cane on the leg of her overstuffed armchair. "Time for dinner!"

Grandma commandeers an escort from amongst the older men and leads him to the dining room through the east door. The adults follow in pairs, while the children and teens exit through the front door to barbecue snags and shrimp in a pit beside the patio. Andy comes over to me to offer his arm, his carefully groomed, handsome face and fit form so attractive in a well-cut tuxedo that my heart skips several beats; I am glad to find that Mrs. Denton has placed him close to her at the head of the table, which we doubled in length, and placed Reggie and me near Gyorgos at the foot.

Opposite Reggie is Geoffrey, whose slender, tow-headed form seems fragile in a dinner suit, and near him are Ruth, Yanni, and Melanie. When everyone is seated, Gyorgos stands and takes several minutes to present his vision for Denton Inn's cuisine and to explain the evening's menu. Then Eva and Bryan bring out the dishes, and Gyorgos encourages us to share the meal family style.

Geoffrey and I have an awkward moment when we realize that Grandma has seated us together because we are both single. She has never accepted that he has no interest in women, or that he prefers animals to humans. He takes her bullying out on me by launching into a description of his methods of collecting semen from studs. Knowing that he is sensitive as well as socially awkward, I am not sure how to respond, and grateful when Gyorgos intervenes. "You're at the table, Geoff, not the trough."

"So how do you rate the cuisine, Georgie?" asks Reggie.

"The skordalia needs work. And we need a few more courses."

A look of angry contempt contorts Yanni's face for a fleeting moment. As I am wondering if I imagined it, he looks straight into my eyes, and seems demonic again for another brief moment. I run the last few days in reverse, wondering what I have done to attract his contempt. I can think of nothing. "Yanni, have I done something wrong?"

"How could you?" he replies with heavy irony. "You do

everything Reg and Gyorgos tell you to."

"I have to admit that your family has changed my life. I've never had it so good, and I'm grateful to all of you."

"And we to you," Reg adds. "You're like a member of the family, now."

"A white sheep to replace the black one," Yanni says.

I am incredulous at Yanni's jealousy. After a confused pause, I ask haltingly, "You mean you?"

"I mean anyone who thinks for himself," Yanni says, fixing wide-open, wild eyes on each member of the family in turn and provoking each and all.

"You're like my studs. They donate sperm, and that's it," Geoffrey says, coming unexpectedly to my defense.

"If Grandma knew about you and Reg ..."

Geoffrey asks in surprise, "Are you and Reggie lickers of the nether lips?"

"They will be if they sit next to you much longer," Melanie says sharply.

Ignoring the others, Ruth tries to rescue me from Yanni's jealousy by saying, "The Greek rellies are more fun. They all talk at once!"

Yanni's energy turns aggressive as he frowns at Reggie. He opens his mouth to say something, but Melanie elbows him and he changes his mind.

The tension and the conversation turn to the cuisine, and to the wines that Reggie selected to go with Gyorgos' new menu. After fielding a variety of opinions, a few of them well thought-out and invaluable to the further development of The Inn, Gyorgos calls for dessert and coffee. When Grandma finishes, she rises and takes the arm of a different elderly gentleman, one who appears unsteady but manages to lead her safely back to the living room.

I walk out with Geoff and then scurry over to Andy, my fellow outsider, who is standing by a back window in the living room. Gyorgos offers a toast to Mrs. Denton in which he compares her to the Queen Mum, while offering her a gin and tonic. Mrs. Denton leans on her cane near the grand piano and listens as her grandson and the other guests take it in turns to offer toasts in her honor. One youngster wishes her another ninety years; Anne recounts a past Christmas party; and so on around the room.

When it's my turn, I say, "To a bold businesswoman!" The guests stare mutely. Apparently I have failed to strike the right note. I fill the silence by saying, "Thanks for including me in your lovely family party."

Mrs. Denton replies sharply, "Reggie wouldn't take no for an answer!"

There is general laughter, from which Reggie attempts to rescue me by saying, "Let's toast Colette on leaving her husband to start a new life!"

"Let's get her down under a real bloke for a change!" Mrs. Denton cackles.

Andy grins and draws the attention onward by giving his toast, "To the most beautiful nonagenarian in Australia!"

Mrs. Denton smiles coyly. By the time the toasts are done, she is in very high spirits, and takes a seat at the piano. She begins by playing Waltzing Matilda, the unofficial national anthem, which everyone sings together and finishes moist-eyed. As Mrs. Denton continues to play, and others to sing, Andy says, "Let's go on walkabout. Leave the family to the family."

"Great idea!"

We go out into the cloudy night and do a circuit of the patio.

I pull my shawl tight against the cold air as we pause to watch the deejay, a teenaged boy with spiky black hair and a studded collar who has set up his turntables and speakers along the south hedge. He is spinning for a wild pack of small boys who are running around a folding table topped with a dimpled ice cream cake. Several girls stand quietly at the table eating cake, but one is running with the boys. She holds a small, barking dog above her head like a winning lottery number. The bursts of her steamy breath fan upward in the cone of light cast by a spotlight on the outside wall of the house. The girl puts down the dog and runs to cut a huge slice of cake; the boys follow.

"There's the next Reg," Andy says. He is standing behind me with his arms crossed against the cold.

"You think she'll ever have kids?"

"A bit late, isn't it?"

"I suppose—I mean I reckon—you're right."

"Grandma likes you, doesn't she?"

"Does she?"

"She wouldn't have teased you like that if she didn't."

"Oh."

"You're like one of these kids. You need everything explained."

"I do. Speaking of which, how are you and Lisa doing?"

Andy's shadow, which stretches beyond the patio, lifts its shoulders into the darkness beyond the hedge. "Unreal. The whole thing's unreal."

"Any regrets?"

"No. Impatient to find out where we'll be, though. It could be months before Lisa can come and live here"

"At least this gives you time to sort things out."

"You like your happy endings, don't you?"

"I treat them as a responsibility. It's our job to watch for opportunities and make endings happy—if we can. Look at Grandma. She's still working at it, and she's ninety! I want to be like that."

Andy's shadow shakes its head.

"You're like that about work," I insist. "Remember how you said you like things to come right at the end of each day?"

"And they do, don't they?"

"Yes. You know how to make it happen every day. I want to be like that."

"Let's walk down to the stable. Reg is already there." Andy turns and leads the way.

We enjoy our rooms in the renovated west stables, and are happy that the horses have moved and relinquished the buildings and yards to humans. While we can still detect notes of straw and leather, as well as of manure and rotting apples, we are now living in compact but elegant luxury. When we reach my room, Andy comes inside as if to continue our conversation and then presses his lips below my ear and whispers, "You need to get under a real bloke, like the lady said."

"It's tempting to imagine how we could comfort each other, but—"

Andy turns my shoulders and kisses me on the mouth. The kiss is tender and delectable and finishes with a firm embrace of urgent need. My thighs feel his firm shanks, and my desire rises to meet his. We kiss again and again, until I hear his belt unbuckle, and feel a silent siren of alarm rise from the small of my back.

I use every particle of self-discipline to push against his powerful chest and look at his face. His eyes are closed. He could be kissing anyone. "Andy, look at me."

The wind stirs a layer of leaf litter outside. My heart aches for his troubles with Lisa. If he and I go on like this, his soul will claim mine and lose hers—and perhaps also his child's.

Andy opens his eyes. His brow builds a furrow of angry frustration.

"If sex is what you need, Andy, why haven't the others satisfied you?"

"I need it from you," he replies glibly.

"Oh, Andy. I love you, I do—as a mate and a brother. So I'm going to try to forget that you want to use my body to avoid learning to deal with your wife and baby."

Andy tenses in fury. His voice holds steady. "We're the same, you and me, hanging on when we should let go. We could help each other. We could take care of each other."

I push resolutely against his warm, inviting chest and feel an urge toward recklessness and risk. "All right, then. I'll call your bluff. If you've really given up on Lisa; if you're ready to stop playing alley cat, and you still want me at the end of Carnival week, and you tell me you want me then the way you're telling me now so that I can feel and believe it, I'll give us a go."

9

Graeme

Early one morning in September, I cross the north pasture under a cloudy sky, avoiding the mass of wool-burdened sheep flowing toward the poplars at the western fence. I smile at the ramshackle pile of metal, wood, and plastic that leans against the makeshift laboratory and the ruined remnant of a stone wall. It is an incubator of fine produce, a muse for Gyorgos' new palette of flavors, but no architect or aesthete gave it a form to reflect its role, and so it appears as the derelict end rather than the fruitful beginning of a grand venture.

I jump the covered trough where Andy is soaking new root-stocks and duck under the plastic flap that serves as door to the hothouse. Inside, the warm, damp air is flavored by compost from kitchen scraps, grass, local grape seeds, worms, and fallen bark. The tomato seedlings are growing delightfully now; their lacy leaves reach several centimeters higher than they did before, and seem to tower over the flats that sit heavily on sawhorse tables. These new green shoots are the center of this Eden, the most beguiling aspect of the miniature farm that is feeding our sweet optimism.

Many of the tomato seedlings are ready for replanting. I roll up my sleeves, select a promising one, ease it out of its flat, and carry it to the spiral stack of planter boxes to press it into an opening in the grainy soil. Intrigued by its earthworm aroma, I place a pinch of soil on my tongue and examine its dry metallic flavor. It is grainy and bitter, richer than the tannic soil of Maine but less layered than the deep, black soil of the Illinois of yester-year. It would have a heartier taste if Gyorgos would let me add manure to his compost. All in good time.

The Inn at Denton is growing so fast that we risk believing the illusion that we can create the new without destroying the old. As yet, we have faced no hard choices. The expansion of the vineyard is limited by nothing but our ability to work. The restaurant is running smoothly for locals on weekends, and will soon be ready for the official launch on Cup Carnival day, when Geoffrey will host a small invitational horse race on the prac-tice track. Yanni has assembled two more yurts for guests, and Geoffrey is training two ponies to enchant city-bred children with country life. If the project succeeds, the family will tear down the hothouse and lab, move the yurts to the south pasture, and erect new structures with stone façades that borrow permanence from geology, tradition from the buildings left by Reggie's ancestors, and culture from art.

For now, everything that we are building is temporary, and in this low season that Reggie describes as fallow, our actions are becoming unfocused and desultory and our souls are absorb-ing an undercurrent of malaise fed by unreconciled differences. Gyorgos has been trying to bolster Reggie's commitment to him by hiring Graeme to offer physical therapy at The Inn, but Reggie has pigeon-holed that plan due to Grandma's efforts to get her to breed. Reggie has been away a lot visiting Graeme, whom she has kept away from the family. Gyorgos has been busy at his city restaurant preparing his top chef for partnership, and for an eventual buyout of Gyorgos' remaining interest. In the absence of these guiding lights, Geoffrey has begun gambling again, and has been spending more and more time at the pub with Andy and Yanni.

In their absence, Melanie and her baby Niko, Ruth and her children, and Lisa and I have become close. This has brought my eclectic faith and practice to Ruth's attention, which has caused her some anxiety about the degree to which Reg and I are non-conformists. Unfortunately, her anxieties that had centered on the worrisome habits of Geoffrey and Yanni are now centered on Reggie's consortship with Graeme, which Ruth views as more sinful than gambling and child neglect. I am now caught between unwanted secrets and the consequences of failing to keep them.

A glass clinks. A shadow moves across the plastic wall that separates the hothouse from the laboratory. It stops in front of the shelf where Reggie keeps her expanding collection of reagents and glassware. I am thrilled that she is here, and can't wait to tell her about today's experimental breakfast of rosehips tea, olives, prunes, and sheep cheese with soft lavasch.

"Hey, Reg! This morning I had arbequina and amfissa olives with prunes!"

"I could never abide arbequina olives!"

"Gyorgos is getting the hang of that sheep cheese, too."

"Those sheep are a bloody nuisance!"

Her tone worries me. "Reg, is Gyorgos pleased with my work?"

"Chefs are bigger prima donnas than winemakers!"

I go to the plastic flap between the laboratory and hothouse and push it open. "Are you okay?"

Reggie is standing at the bench holding a dark brown bottle

filled with a reagent she uses to test the soil. She puts it down, wipes her brow with her wrist, and clasps her grubby hands like a supplicant. "Grandma's called a family meeting tonight. I tried to keep you and Andy well out of it, but there'll be hell to pay for all of us now that Ruth knows about Graeme."

This is the first time I have seen Reggie tense. "I'm sorry," I confess. "I was my usual open self with Ruth and got to like and trust her. I didn't realize how intolerant she could be. And I should tell you now that even though I know it's not my place, and even though I regret telling her about my life—and with mine, yours—I just can't abide secrets."

Reggie's face slackens in shock. "You told her?"

"I'm sorry. I told her about my celibacy practice, and then that you had taught me. And one time I mentioned Graeme teaching you sacred sex."

Reggie nods. She starts to speak and then stops, and then starts again. "I should have warned you not to tell her. Ack! This is awful, just awful. Grandma can be spot-on, but sometimes she's mad! Her interference could be the beginning of the end."

"Goodness, Reg. That's portentous. Can't you just stand up to Ruth?"

Reggie sighs. "I will try. But it may not work, in which case it won't be your fault or mine for living and loving openly. It'll be the right solution for the situation."

"There's only one thing to do if Grandma doesn't like it, and that's to whack Mrs. Elizabeth Denton with that cane," I say.

Reggie doesn't laugh, but she takes a deep breath, puts her hands over her face, and lets out a self-mocking growl. "I have to go and fetch him for tonight's meeting. Will you come with me?"

"I'd like that. Especially given that my peacemaking skills are useless in the absence of people who believe in peace."

A breeze rattles the plastic walls of the laboratory. Outside, a sheep bleats like a crying baby. I bring my palms together in front of my heart to signal support, and we stand in the uncertain, creative nexus of East and West, between old and new, barrenness and fecundity of all kinds, womanhood and elderhood, fertility and wisdom, completion and continuation.

"Will we be coming to dinner?"

"No. I already explained the situation to Gyorgos. He's going to make a traditional Greek meal, and Mum will take your place as his sous-chef. We can grab a bite after Grandma goes up to bed."

Reggie sighs deeply. I lift a bucket from the floor and add fresh water to the antique floral washbasin on the counter. She leans over to scrub her nails with a splayed brush, which reveals her profile in silhouette against the sunlit gap in the far plastic wall. The skin under her chin is loosening. Age and trouble are coming to call, and are leaving their marks on us. I once thought that consort practice could solve one's life problems and keep one young, but now I see it as a way to take on more responsibility. As we empty the basin onto the planters and start across the pasture to the great house, I return to the vision of giving birth to partnership and community rather than to a child. There are already many too many Connollys on my father's side and Landrys on my mother's, and far too few groups that explore the unselfish, unbounded creation of new ways of life that suit times when childbearing is a choice.

I say as bracingly as I can, "Remember our fantasy of setting up a winery, restaurant, and retreat center someplace else? I could cater for it. If things don't work out here, maybe you and Andy and Graeme and I could do that. What do you think?"

"I don't know." Her eyes, which are as vague and gray as the horizon, pore over the earth ahead of us. "Right now I can't think of starting anything." After a few minutes, she says, "I'm heartened that you've continued your celibacy practice, though."

"How so?"

"You've been showering Andy with love and compassion free of desire. It's driving him mad—and it's changing him."

"I think we're beginning to synergize without sex, but we use it all for work. You said you and Graeme use your energy for a purpose. Like what?"

"Sometimes we use it to develop skills like strength, clarity, or compassion, and sometimes we send it to his group, or to someone in need. He does other things that I don't really understand. He's explained it, but I don't have the experience to grasp it."

"Does he ever give the energy to you?"

"Ah, yeah, especially during harvest, but most often we give and receive in equal measure. In ancient times adepts used their energy to strengthen the boundaries around a family or tribe. Now we use it to dissolve them, and to protect life on earth."

"I wish we could do that with Ruth."

"It isn't easy to be effective. A tantrika has to have very pure intentions and finely honed skills. And when you become effective, it isn't all that easy to be safe. A clumsy beginner or a malicious adept can break a mind, cause illness, or draw someone else's strength. Graeme could do it with my help, but it wouldn't change Ruth's dogma, and Gyorgos is too strong-minded."

"I'd like to learn to do it right, and to find a consort."

"I suppose now that the secret is out, Graeme and I could give some classes. Melanie and Yanni could use them, and so could some of our Uni friends."

"If you do, I'd like to be part of it."

"I'm most worried about Laura and Clive," she says, referring to their starving artist friends from Uni. "He went to India and came back broken, with no idea what happened or how to restore himself. I suspect that he came into contact with a guru who took too much of his energy, possibly intentionally."

"How can someone take energy without permission?"

Reggie snorts. "Many people are wide open—you, for instance. Graeme could have you for breakfast. But he wouldn't. For one thing, he has me."

Reggie stops to pull dead leaves from an old vine, revealing green ones underneath. We pause at the edge of the Denton yard so that Reggie can finish her final point. "Leaders do tantra all the time without knowing it. It's the hidden source of power behind professional organizations, priests, universities, corporations. It comes naturally, like the meditative practice you used to do in your armchair in Maine. The trouble with most leaders is that they feed the group ego rather than feeding its spirit."

"So, for you tantra is another word for energetics, for practices that draw on—or feed—the energy body."

"Yes, in a way. Energetics fuels it. As you say, in people who desire concord, and in adepts who work purposefully rather than inadvertently or secondarily."

As we lope down to the stables to bathe and put on our city clothes, I make a mental note to try and feed the shared spirit of those of us motivated to nurture The Inn. After, when we walk out to the side yard, the tiny yellow ball of the sun is beginning to penetrate the gray haze. It is easy to see that the light will soon emerge clear and bright, and that the gum-scented breeze that is riffling and stroking the spring-green grass will soon coax out new growth. It is not easy to see what is possible for us, or what we will become. I hold out my palms to catch the breeze within the breeze, the river of Life in which we have our being and with which we aim to live well.

Reggie goes to Gyorgos' shiny, black sedan, takes the driver's seat, and slams the door. I take the passenger seat to her left, which is sticky with children's handprints. "Why your brother's car?"

"The back seat is more comfortable."

When we gain the road, I point out the budburst that is touching radically pruned spurs with new evidence of rebirth, but Reggie is quiet, and I let her be. I watch the birds gleaning and the fields greening, the sun clearing the heavens to let in the light of spring. Many miles later, when we become mired in sluggish traffic in the revitalizing suburb of North Melbourne, Reggie sighs and then laughs. "Ah, right. It's the day of the Grand Final."

"The what?"

"The last game of the footy season, the one that decides the premiership. Look at the fans!"

We roll past families and couples and teenagers in white and blue scarves and hats. In front of us, a boisterous group at a bus stop darts daringly out in front of our car and then staggers back to the curb. At a stoplight, a derelict leans against a pub window and points at us, shouting angry insults at the Sydney Swans. A group of hoarse young men chant a semi-hostile attack. Apparently our lack of colors is enough to brand us as the enemy.

It is well after noon when Reggie turns into a street lined with trees and California-style red brick houses. She parks by a half-front that has green and white trim and a red-tiled roof. Its yard is barely tended, and its painted steps look worn and neglected. I follow her in through the side door, realizing that even though

I have seen Graeme I haven't thought of him as a therapist who makes housecalls in suburbia. Once inside, Reggie takes off her shoes and pads up a long hall to a bright front room.

A scratchy bass voice says, "Come in, Colette."

I go into the white-painted front room that is dominated by a bay window and heavy wood trim. The golden wood floor provides warm visual contrast. My eyes find Graeme, who is sitting perfectly still in a threadbare armchair. His closely trimmed black beard and receding hairline frame his huge brown eyes. His gaze is so intense that I instinctively pull up my jacket collar. Then I sense his ocean of calm, and I relax into it. His hands are smooth and thick and well groomed. Perfect for a physiotherapist, a body worker who does many kinds of hands-on treatments.

Reggie sits in an armchair opposite Graeme's. Between them is a huge, sheepskin-covered hospital chair with gadget-covered armrests and a reclining back. I finally notice a pair of wide, gray-green eyes staring out of the bony relic of a woman's face. She has thick, wavy blond hair, and her pale body is laid out on the chair like a deflated sex doll. Her gaze reminds me of an octopus staring out of an aquarium.

"Oh. Hello."

"Collo, why don't you take a seat on the sofa?" Graeme says.

I pull my eyes away from hers and step backward to plop onto the shiny chintz sofa. Behind me, a high table holds a huge television set, a mass of electronic equipment, and stacks of dusty videotapes. When I sit, I become a part of the entertainment system, and feel put on the spot. I wonder why I am not more distressed and then realize that the room is like a love-bath. This time, Reggie is not the only source of sweetness; Graeme also radiates kindness and warmth. He strokes his beard with his right knuckle. "My visits give Trudi and her caregiver a bit of respite. He should be back soon."

"I feel like I'm being interrogated by The Trinity," I say with a half-smile. The others laugh. Graeme says, "Trudi likes a joke."

When a burly-haired man with black stubble enters, Reg, Graeme, and I take our leave. I get in the back seat of the car, Reggie in the drivers' seat, and Graeme in the seat beside her. Trudi's eyes were lively, and yet it feels as if we have emerged from a tomb. A voice in my heart asks: *How long will she be alive? How long will we?*

Soon, we are speeding north on Punt Street through a neighborhood laced with railroad tracks. Here the streets are lined with old, finely-crafted Victorian homes and recently renovated brick warehouses. The area we reach next appears neglected but is enlivened by families in bush hats and shoe boots who are streaming away from the massive oval of Melbourne Cricket Ground, which comes into view at the far end of a grassy strip to our left. We stop at a wide intersection with shelters on each corner where throngs of red- and white-hatted families are standing quietly, their faces miserable. The driver of the car beside us honks at them; its occupants are waving blue and white scarves out of open windows.

"The Roos must have taken the premiership," Graeme says.

"Andy'll be happy," Reggie replies.

As we drive north into the countryside to the Dividing Range, the day turns to dusk. Scattered gums shiver in brief gusts. We meld into a trio that harmonizes silently and invisibly. As we approach Denton, the mood breaks and Reg says sadly, "Our partnership's none of Grandmas's bizzo!"

"When you're ninety, I reckon everyone else seems daft," Graeme notes placidly. "And change gets hard. You can reassure Grandma; Collo can help with that."

Reggie sighs. "Grandma's always liked you. I don't blame her for being angry with me for keeping you away."

"I'm glad to be coming up with you. I like Grandma and I can help with Ruth."

"I hope so."

As we pass through the front gate of Denton Stables, we seem to breach the wall that has separated Reggie's two lives. I feel relieved and say so. Reggie parks in back, and we come around to enter the front door together. Inside, the new podium light on the U-shaped reception desk illuminates the reservation book that lays open beneath it. The tables are set for dinner, and the living room is brightly lit behind the closed French doors.

"Is that you, Victoria Regina?" calls Grandma's scratchy voice from the top of the staircase. As her cane begins to thump down the dark stairs, Reggie rushes up to take her arm, and Grandma adds, "Colette, go fetch Melanie!"

I rush out the door and navigate the familiar ruts of the dirt track that leads to the south stable, which Geoffrey is sharing with Yanni's family. I find Melanie waiting upstairs in a lounge room.

As we hurry back up the track together, Melanie says, "Ruth's upset."

When we reach the grassy slope, we hear shouting in the distant kitchen and the banging of pots and pans. "Sounds like Gyorgos isn't too happy, either!"

Inside the foyer, we exchange glances of semi-mock terror before entering the living room and closing the curtained French doors behind us. Grandma is doddering in front of the cold hearth in a loose brown shift, leaning on her cane and eyeing Reg and Graeme, who sit in padded wooden chairs to Grandma's left. Ruth is sitting in an armchair with her back to us, wearing a bright fuscia robe that dominates the old and faded décor. Anne sits on the settee opposite the hearth, knitting placidly between sips of herbal tea. She appears at first glance to be as relaxed and composed as ever, but her eyes, which are superfluous to the task of her skilled hands, are observing Grandma with concern and Ruth with skeptical displeasure. Melanie takes the open seat beside Anne, and I sit beside Melanie. Grandma ignores me, which I take as acceptance into the circle of family women.

She dodders toward Graeme and gives his leg a whack with her cane and asks him haughtily, "What do you have to say about this horizontal dancing with Reggie?"

Graeme says, "It's the sacred heart of our lives."

Grandma looks at Reg in surprise, and then laughs with the "ah, ah, ah" sound that ends in a coughing fit.

Ruth pulls her feet up on the seat cushion and puts her arms around her knees. Anne sighs and leans over her knitting with an unreadable expression that is her facsimile of equanimity, and that may have offset the explosive character of Reggie's absent father, who is said to have expressed the strong emotions that they shared.

"What do you know about this?" Grandma suddenly says to me. "Are you a part of this? Speak up! And don't think you can talk around me. I've got my hearing aid turned on!"

"I also keep an eclectic—and unusual—system of faith and practice. For me, it's part of conscious living."

Grandma frowns. "No clergy?"

"No. And no avoiding responsibility."

"Suits me. What's the problem?" Grandma asks, thumping Ruth with her cane.

"The Bible says that … it's … wrong … pagan …" Ruth's voice trails off.

Pivoting abruptly, and nearly losing her balance in the process, Grandma pounds her cane on the hearth. "You are each responsible for your own way of life."

Reggie glances at Ruth, who stares at the floor.

Grandma turns to Graeme and asks, "What do you do now?"

Graeme tells her. She says, "Something useful. Good. You can stay and take care of me while we figure out what to do about the two of you. Do you plan to marry and have children?"

Graeme says, "No, Grandma. Our lives are full. Reg likes to refresh our commitment every time we meet, and she doesn't want children."

Grandma slumps sadly.

Graeme adds gently, "And I have clients in town who need me."

"You can drive from here," Anne declares.

"They could live in one of Yanni's yurts," offers Melanie.

Ruth looks up and adjusts her position, which reveals a rosary clasped in her hand. I wonder if her faith came from the outside in, or the inside out, and whether she feels obliged to take non-conformity as a threat to the orthodoxy she works to demonstrate. Thoughts and feelings cause her expression to vacillate between love and fear. Finally she says, "I can see that this has been hard on you both. Why don't you stay here together and see how it goes?"

Melanie says uneasily, "Yanni won't like it."

"I reckon you're right," Reggie concurs. "He opposes the

mixing of religion with sexuality or spirituality. And he seems to be getting more and more impulsive and explosive."

"He misses his mates at Bell's Beach and his surfing. I'm not sure … that he'll stay."

Ruth sighs heavily. "I shouldn't judge. I can see that you're loving and committed. And it would be good for the children to have another dependable man at the stables."

"Well?" Grandma asks sharply.

"Thank you, Grandma. I'll stay." Graeme says. "And Ruth can let us know how she feels about it."

Grandma says, "Good. Take me up."

Reggie and I exchange glances. I put my hand over my heart in a gesture of love and hope.

10

Confusion

Two weeks later, Andy snaps a photo of me. He says that I look beautiful in it; it's true that I felt content and the photo shows it. In the photo, I am sitting on a patio chair in a white shirt, slacks, and apron, leaning back on my hands, with one leg drawn up, a strand of hair straying from my chef's hat, eyes bright with a smile. My fingers are covered with small cuts and my palms and forehead are damp, but that doesn't show and didn't matter because I'd found my vocation and become mates with Reggie and Andy and friends with all but Yanni.

Soon, I am helping to prepare a buffet that will present new recipes for the grand opening of The Inn at Denton, an invitation-only event. We are listening to distant music rather than conversing, and we speak only when we deviate from established ritual, as when Gyorgos teaches me to make a white sauce for his new canapés of nori-topped shiitake pastitsio on rice crackers. Because I have made many white sauces, I am impatient with his instruction until he teaches me something new, how to add lemon without spoiling the texture.

I am able now to go from one task to another so as to ensure that everything will come together at the right time. I set out blocks of cheese surrounded by arcs of crackers to make a floral pattern on a large glass platter; heat plates; cool glasses; make centerpieces of spring flowers; and carve butter curls. When the first course is ready, I stay in the kitchen, where I drizzle raspberry coulis on chilled dessert plates, fill cannoli shells with pre-prepared raspberry mousse, and plate them with small scoops of fresh lemon sorbet. After I finish, I put the plates on the dessert cart and roll it into the dining room.

When the luncheon is finished and we have eaten and cleaned up, I take a break and walk toward the south pasture. As I rub together my finely cut, garlicky hands for heat, I am delighted to see Reg striding up to the patio from the direction of the practice track. Delight turns to dismay when I realize her face is radiating upset. I put my hands on my heart and prepare my body to do what it can do to hold us steady.

"What's the matter?" I ask when she is within ten feet.

"It's Yanni, the little prat! He doesn't think about anyone but himself! He's invited everyone here for Cup Day, and told them about my private class in tantric sex!"

"I know."

In my mind's eye, I see Yanni standing at the bar in Andy's favorite pub, ordering drinks for everyone in the place. He invites them to the class, and Andy teases me, saying that going there with me will be his reward for staying in nights. Those who are sharing pints near us seem lightly amused. I see no sign of shock or offense, and little sign of interest or titillation.

"Why didn't you tell me?"

"I was at the pub when he invited everyone to the class. They seemed to take it as a joke. I didn't think he'd done any harm."

"You don't understand; he's inviting everyone to the dinner, and to the fancy dress party, and to my class—and to his porn party. He knows we distinguish between sacred and profane sex, and he's trying to profane our practice, to make it like his. There's no telling what he'll do, except that he'll probably try to sabotage everything that we've all been working for."

"Are you worried that he'll put off Gyorgos' investors?"

Reggie throws back her head. "Ugh! I hadn't thought of that. Thank God we scheduled the grand opening dinner on the Friday night before Cup Day!"

"We're probably the only people in miles who think that either tantra or sex might be sacred. Who could Yanni confuse who isn't confused already?"

"The Plymouth Brethren, for starters. Some of Yanni's childhood mates are part of a Millennialist splinter group. The elders have very specific ideas about theology, and they won't want their kids exposed to Hindu or Buddhist teachings, especially not secret mantra. And they certainly won't countenance any outside ideas or practices related to sex."

"Why don't you call off the class?" I ask.

After a pause, Reggie replies sadly, "Dutchy asked me to do the session for the sake of her family, and so did Clive and Melanie. I reckon her invitation triggered Yan's hostility, but I don't want to let them down."

"Can you move the class to a secret location?"

"Yes! We'll make it strictly private and hold it away from the party."

"That should protect the class, at least."

"Let's hope so," she says.

"I find all of this pointless conflict terribly confusing. I thought I had developed a worldview that could accommodate malice and caprice, but the flow of events is too complex, too unpredictable. It's easier to assume chaos, which is neither redemptive nor destructive."

"Look, complexity entails hazard and surprise. All we can do is set our intentions to respond as wisely as we can on the spot, and to remember that everything is uncertain. That's different to confusion."

"Then why do I feel confused?" I ask with a laugh.

Reggie stands still for a moment, eyes closed. "I talked with Graeme. He'd be happy to partner you for the class, if you're ready."

I feel a frisson of dread on my nape. "Who would sit with you?"

"I might invite Joe." Reggie is referring to their ever-gloomy, ne-'er-do-well single friend from university.

That doesn't feel right. "Do you think it's a good idea?"

"Graeme could be your teacher, and I could be Joe's. You could avoid the harm that might come of sitting with Andy. Graeme could even initiate you sexually. He hasn't done it in years, but he might do it if I asked him, and if he thought you were ready."

"Oh, Reg, please don't. I love you like a sister and I wouldn't risk that for anything. And—to be blunt—I wouldn't want to have sex with him even if I didn't know you."

"He'd only do it if you were both ready."

How could he know? I didn't want to know this. I don't want to think of you like this. "I must not be ready. The thought of doing that makes me very sad. I see your bond as sacred and wouldn't want to come between you two—or lose track of my conscience."

"Our traditions include sexual initiation."

"I don't want to include it in mine. It would probably unhinge me."

"I respect that, but I'd encourage you to think about your reasons."

"How are you and Graeme holding up right now?"

"Graeme'll be all right; he's very strong. But Yanni's draining us. I almost wish he had made up his mind to leave us."

"I saw him whipping one of the horses yesterday. He was out of control."

"He's angry, and he's taking it out on everyone and everything. I wish I could persuade Gyorgos to ask Yan to leave, but Gyorgos is determined to tame Yan."

As I return to the kitchen, I realize that Denton Inn could fail even as we work toward the debut dinner to which Gyorgos has invited the most influential people he knows, including food critics, restaurateurs, and investors. I struggle to concentrate, and I cut my finger badly. At the earliest opportunity, I hang up my apron and hat and exit through the foyer, where Andy is standing at the reception desk leaning on his elbows, perusing his open newspaper.

I pause to ask, "Any news for me?"

"No, but I got plenty *from* you," he replies, with a grin. "You and Reg ought to find a more private place to natter."

"What did you hear?"

Andy folds the paper and puts it under his arm, and then comes around the desk to walk out the front door with me. "I heard you were invited to a class and didn't want to go with Graeme."

Andy and I walk past the yurts and down to the stable, over hollows of rocks and grass where shadows pool like liquid night. We cheer ourselves with talk of the Roos' premiership, and the latest gossip from the pub where Andy has his daily pint. They are abuzz with the news of Geoffrey's gambling withdrawal and of his plans for the first Annual Denton Cup, which is only one of many in the area but is attracting attention because it signals the resurgence of an important stud farm. The neighbors are also watching Gyorgos' restaurant with keen anticipation, hoping that he will draw well-heeled customers on weekends, and so create new jobs.

They are also spreading lurid rumors about Reggie and Yanni's perversions. Andy mocks them and tells them they've watched too much porn, but that only feeds their fun. Reggie is right; Yanni may draw a tabloid-ready circus to The Inn now— or on Cup Day. He has put the whole project at risk. When we reach the top landing, I am in danger of slipping into pessimism about Denton's future. Andy stops, presses his body against mine, and pushes me against the wall in the shadows. I smell stale ale and bread on his breath. He whispers in my ear, "I know what I want. But what do you want? What are your dreams now?" I can't see the expression on his shadowed face, but I can hear an unaccustomed absence of irony in his voice.

"I want you to want Lisa. I like her. She just needs time. As for me, I have a vocation, which is a blessing, and I still hope to co-found a community with you and Reg and your partners someday."

Andy brushes his fingertips across my nape and kisses me sweetly on the cheek. My body responds to his caress like an opening flower. In the flurry leading up to the opening, I have been neglecting my celibacy practice. He says, "Reg's class is for lovers, not strangers; let her look after Graeme, and let me look after you. Call my bluff?"

I gasp. "Can you look after me?"

"You can count on me."

Andy backs away until his beguiling body is illuminated by the cone of light. I bolt into my room and dive under the covers like a child seeking safety. I touch my cheek where he kissed it and realize that I do trust him, and that I yearn to count on him. But he is not my match, and I am not his. I am sliding into a fantasy that undermines our intentions, and so losing my grip on what matters most. I am losing faith in the family, and I fear isolation. Andy seems ready to compromise, but it feels forced. I must hold our dreams. I must pull clarity from confusion.

I hop out of bed into the chill of darkness and hurry to Reg's room, where I knock on her door. As I wait, I realize that Graeme may be with her, or they may both be gone. As I turn away, the door opens and Reg is standing within, wrapped in a towel, dripping.

"Sorry to intrude," I say. "Can I talk to you about Andy and me?"

Reg smiles broadly. "Sure. Come in. There's no better time to refresh our practices." Reggie and I sit on the floor and adjust our posture. We send our ear and eye energy down our central channels and move our focus to important centers of energy that refresh my celibacy and increase our vitality. Later, in bed, I relax into my familiar, preternatural peace.

11

Carnival

At nine o'clock on the first Tuesday of November, after the wildly successful opening of The Inn at Denton, I look forward to my first Melbourne Cup Day and the first race at Denton Stables in more than a decade. I wait inside the front door of the big stone house with camera in hand. The family will be gathering for a picture before leaving for Flemington Race Course. As long-time members of the Victoria Racing Club, they will have excellent seats with prime views of the horses, and a good pole position for the race for best ladies' hat.

Though I will be staying behind with Gyorgos to help him with the catering, I too have caught Cup Carnival fever, and am thrilled when Reggie descends the stairs like a Ziegfeld girl in an emerald green dress and a white hat with asymmetric brim and a high spray of peacock feathers. I take a photo of her, and of Anne, who comes down in a bright blue tailored suit with a matching top hat that shows off her pale eyes. The three of us applaud and I snap a photo when Ruth, Melanie, and Grandma come down the stairs wearing matching vintage cloches from the sultry forties.

"Is that your lucky hat, Grandma?" Reggie asks.

"I've worn it every year since our Knight Errantry took the Cup and earned a lot of lucre in stud fees."

I wish I'd bet on Lisa for best hat when I see her coming up the front walk wearing a boxy pink hat with sheer stripes. Behind her come the men in their suits, Graeme sturdy in a slick black tuxedo, Yanni electrifying in white tails, and Andy dashing in splashy shades of blue and gray.

Geoffrey, the lone resident of Denton Stables who hasn't bet in the family's Cup race pool—or in any pool organized by friends or neighbors—is suffering through Cup week like a recovering alcoholic at a cocktail party. To my surprise, Yanni, who has taken on the role of family bookie, has given me long odds that Geoffrey will lapse and punt before Sunday. Now Geoffrey stands at the podium looking like an idle Maître De until I take his arm and lead him to the front steps for a group photo.

"You're the beautiful people! Who knew?"

"You haven't seen the best of it," Andy replies with a wink.

I am so proud of the good looks of my adoptive family that I take many photos on the steps, and then lure them into the foyer to take their portrait in the restaurant. I take pictures until Yanni can't hold still anymore. I hope they may prolong the anticipation by opening a bottle of bubbly, but Grandma leads them straight out to the cars. Anne follows with Reg, and the rest follow en masse, and so get momentarily stuck in the door and have to jockey for position. I stand on the patio and enjoy the sun that is shining through a thin haze while one by one the cars speed up the drive.

When the cars have disappeared and the dust of the drive has settled, I feel uneasy. Everything looks slick. Everyone is dressed as if eager to put a good face on something that they can't trust. I wonder if it's just me feeling left out, or if others feel uneasy as well. Like secrets, buried conflicts tend to draw darkness around them and so to become more deeply hidden even as they become more dire. I can see why Grandma desires Reggie's grandchildren; that undeniable sign of future hope draws light and love, and transforms brooding resentments into warmth that drives cooperation. Except, it seems, in Yanni's case. His love for his baby son is like his love for his wife, like quicksilver; changeable, unreliable, and—apparently—forgettable.

Joy is evident in the children's races at the practice track, which turn out to be a big success. Even Laura and Clive's skateboarding larrikins canter happily around the track. Best of all, Gyorgos gets a call from an old school friend who came to Friday's grand opening dinner and who has decided to invest heavily in The Inn. Gyorgos will have the capital to convert the house into a luxurious inn with fine dining, a new guest wing, a signature wine label, spa services, and saddle-riding and skateboarding programs, and flying fox lines for families who come up for the school holidays. Rather than make him happy and carefree, however, the news intensifies his ambition; he takes the time to give his team a talk that presses us to reach a higher level of excellence.

As I dice onions, I wipe my eyes on my white linen coat and ask, "Gyorgos?"

"Yes, Colette," he replies absently as he halves a freshly plucked chicken.

"Will your guests be staying for the fancy dress party?"

"They've all returned to Melbourne."

"I'm planning to dress as a nun. I hope that won't offend anyone."

"That depends entirely on your comportment!"

During my break, I discover that although rain left muddy

rivulets in the trails, the cool gusts that followed raise fine grit that feels like sandpaper on bare legs. I circle the house to the leeward side, from which vantage point I can safely watch the cars as they arrive. An unfamiliar truck rolls down the drive pulling a shiny brown horse trailer with a lightning logo. The hidden horse will undoubtedly participate in the official Denton race, the winner of which will take home a tarnished cup of unknown provenance that Melanie found in the attic. I return to the kitchen and assemble a platter of marinated meat and vegetable kebabs for Bryan and Eva to grill at the track, where Yanni has filled the huge white tent with food and drinks tables as well as seating for guests.

For the next several hours, Gyorgos and I and the staff that he hired for the day focus all of our attention on the catering for the race, the afternoon snacks, and the Greek–Italian dinner that Gyorgos planned as a break from his Greek–Asian fusion cuisine. Only when a car door slams outside do I realize that I have missed both the Melbourne Cup and Denton Cup races. I put down my pan and run to the foyer to ask who has won, and then stop in surprise. A crowd of unfamiliar people is mingling in the foyer, all talking at once.

"What's going on?" I ask Melanie, who is standing near the kitchen door.

"Grandma's invited the guests for sherry. Didn't Gyorgos tell you?"

"No!" I step aside as a harried girl breezes past me to put a tray on a linen-clad table on the front patio. "He's got several teams going, and he's using me as the kitchen floater, doing whatever he wants me to at the moment."

"When will you be free?"

"I'll join you for dinner, and for the fancy dress party."

"See you at eight on the patio?"

"Right-o. It'll be strange and wonderful to leave the kitchen!"

Melanie tells me that Saintly has won the Melbourne Cup, which means I lost my bet in the family pool. And, to everyone's surprise, Emily's horse won the Denton Cup, and everyone but Louis lost. I give Melanie a hug and return to the kitchen, where I think of nothing but cooking until my next break, when I go out to the patio again to enjoy its view of the land.

The wind has died down. Late afternoon sun is filtering through the western stand of poplars, painting lacy murals of light on the yurts across the drive. Geoffrey is leading Gyorgos' children down a bridle path toward the practice track and its huge, white-painted canvas tent. Taki, who is riding one of the ponies, is talking, as usual. When he turns in the saddle to shout at his brother, he spooks a kangaroo family grazing on the south hill and flushes a flock of Major Mitchell's pink cockatoos from the trees by the house. The farm is alive with the hard work and creative spirit of its industrious family, and seems more beautiful and lively today than ever before. My heart opens cautiously to hope.

Reggie's friends approach from the practice track. I hurry down to greet Roger and Judy, who will be joining Louis and Emily and Laura and Clive in a guest yurt. After a complex dance of hugs and kisses, we succeed in hauling their luggage down to the far yurt. Laura and Clive's spindly teenaged boys seem resolutely resentful at first, but they brighten with kindness when they see Emily's three little girls, who are anxious about staying away from home. The boys go gaga over the girls' voluptuous babysitter. The young people form a tribe and take turns spreading out their doonas on the floor of a plain but comfortable room. Before they are settled, and while the babysitter is organizing a trek down to the bluff, I run up to the kitchen and work at making sauces and plating dishes. After a couple of hours, Gyorgos dismisses me and admonishes me to wear my costume well.

I walk down to the stables to dress. The sun is already setting, but it will be over an hour before Melanie and I are to meet on the patio. I take my time dressing for dinner, beginning with a bath and a luxurious grooming, and a stroll to watch the twilight fade and the stars come out.

I am not worried now about what is to come; I am only curious. The successful debut of Gyorgos' restaurant, my increasing mastery of cooking, and the deepening group-mind that I share with Reggie, Andy, Lisa, and Graeme are memories that I will cherish, but Reggie is right: whatever we lose now will have been too weak to last. I trust that while Yanni may do serious damage to the family and its business at any time, but the blessings that we have co-created here are threads that we will carry forward in one form or another; any curses are threads that will break and be left behind.

When the time is near, I put on a black slip dress and silver earrings and carry my silver sandals in hand; I slip on my boots for the walk up to the patio. I walk slowly in the darkness, but am still the first to arrive. I attempt to behave as a guest, but soon run to fetch a kitchen scissor and then nip up to the main road to gather sprigs of jasmine and return to decorate the drinks table.

As I stand back to look at the arrangement, Andy's voice asks, "Are you decorating a dunny?"

Reggie laughs and teases, "Are those your shoes for the fancy dress party?"

As Reggie and her family step up onto the patio with Andy, I pull off my boots and put on my sandals. "The patio has all the softness of a quarry."

Reggie puts a hand on the orange lily that is about to fall from behind her ear and leans back to look up at the stone walls. "You know, Grandma used to have an arbor beyond the hedge, and umbrellas for the tables."

"I'll talk with Gyorgos about that," Ruth says, pulling up her fuchsia shawl.

"Should we do anything more to prepare?" I ask.

"Reconceive!" Reggie laughs and raises her hands in imitation of Gyorgos. "I'm joking. It's time to relax. Even Gyorgos is dining with us tonight!"

"Where were you?"

"Watching the last races at the practice track. It's been great fun."

As Andy selects a cold lager from the ice-filled esky and Ruth asks Reggie about the wine offerings, Melanie pulls me to one side of the patio. She looks over her shoulder to make sure we are alone and then whispers, "I heard you might sleep with Andy tonight."

"Sleep with him? We once talked of going to Reggie's class."

"But how will you feel when he sleeps with someone else? Lisa doesn't seem to care."

"Goodness. I'd feel worse if he left her for me."

"What if you two don't want to work together after you sleep together?"

"Why do you think we will?"

"Yanni's told everyone that Andy was chuffed that you'd finally agreed to sleep with him on Cup Day."

"I only promised to call his bluff, not to—well—we talked about the possibility, and he said he knows what he wants ... but it feels like a joke that's got out of control."

"You should know that Yan's taken bets on whether you and Andy will go to Reggie's sessions together."

"What?"

"Most people bet that you won't. They see Andy as a bit of a knocker, and you as the kind who can say no to him."

"Well. At least there's that. Did you bet that I'd go with him?"

"Yes."

I stand with my mouth open. I am in shock and feel unpleasantly exposed and guilty, which is probably just what Yanni wanted. I watch Melanie smile and squeeze my free hand and walk away, and try to regain my poise and prepare to laugh off the inevitable teasing.

Ruth approaches, drawing up her shawl. "This is a big day for Gyorgos. I hope you had your mind on your work."

"Has Gyorgos said anything bad about my work?"

"He says you've been distracted lately."

Ruth is leaning forward with her eyes and mouth open, scanning my face like a woman thirsty for gossip. "Don't worry Ruth, the apprenticeship is my number one priority."

"Yanni's bringing someone for you."

"What? Thanks for the heads up. I'll make a point of ignoring his tricks."

I turn and head for the drinks table and nearly run into Roger. "So," he says, taking a swig from a stubby of bitters, "I hear you're developing your culinary artistry, now, doll."

His wife Judy adds warmly, "I didn't think you'd advance so quickly. Good on ya!"

"How about Andy, then?" Rog says, taking a swig of beer.

"Andy?"

"I hear he fancies you. Do you fancy him?"

"Well, I like him very much, and he's a mate, but he's married."

"Ah, look, Andy only married so as to be unavailable for matrimony."

"He's always been available nights, hasn't he?" Judy asks, stroking Rog's chest. "He's perfect if you fancy a fling."

"I don't," I say awkwardly, standing on tiptoes to look at the drinks table, where I spot Reggie. "It's so good to see you. I look forward to sitting with you at dinner."

I dart over to the drinks table and take Reggie's arm, and then maneuver to the edge of the patio and take Andy's. I draw them down the curving walk. I tell them about the betting pool; both laugh. I ask, "What should we do?"

"I should bet that we'll go, and then we should go. Lisa and I could use the money," Andy says.

"If no one specified how long you had to stay to win, you could just come and sit and stare at each other and leave. We start with gazing," Reg says.

"How would Lisa feel about that?" I ask Andy.

"She'll be all right. But I'll tell her you asked."

Reg laughs and then shakes her head. "It'd be a shame if Yan got the best of us."

"True. All right. I'm in."

I go to the kitchen, assemble an antipasto platter from the most select preserves, and engage two idle servers in preparing a cart of pastries and coffee for dessert. As I wheel the cart into the dining room, Emily and Louis come to walk me to Reggie's table and to ask, "So, how are you and Andy getting on?"

"Don't tell me you're going to place a bet!"

Emily replies, "We did already. We're only concerned about your welfare now, but we needn't be! You look beautiful, and I hear that you're becoming a wonderful chef."

"You know, Collo," Louis says, eying me thoughtfully before gallantly pulling my chair out and then pushing it in when I sit down, "Yanni started taking bets on you and a bloke by the name of Hawk. Do you know anything about that?"

I groan. "I heard that Yanni's bringing someone for me— maybe that's Hawk?"

Embarrassment and confusion overtake me. I eat quickly, without entering into the conversation, and then bolt for the stables. Unfamiliar noises, some of which come from the main house and patio and some from the yurts and stables, disorient me in the dark. Unfamiliar faces pass. I realize that it is close to Halloween, when the dead were said to leave their graves. The casual sadomasochism of Yanni's betting pool no longer seems like boyish foolery. I worry that Yanni's friend—or even Andy—may be possessed by the shadows and do something rash. I worry that I might.

In my room, I wash at the basin and put on the nun costume that I rented in St. Kilda, partly as a joke and partly as penance for having been angry at nuns for far too long. When I have made my way through the night in my black habit and white-edged cowl, I see that most of the other partygoers are dressed more for a carnival than for an American Halloween party. I feel silly in my habit, until I return to the house and spot Dutchy in the dining room wearing a folk dress with wooden clogs.

Through the open French doors, those of us crowding into the foyer can see the deejay spinning techno music, jerking his arms from the turntables to the flashing lights and fog machine and back again. Liz and Veronica, both dressed as fan dancers in pasties and thongs, are struggling with unwieldy fans of emu feathers. Louis, who is dressed like the Red Baron, is dancing with Emily, who is dressed as a flapper. Geoffrey, more attractive than usual in rock glam makeup and temporary tattoos, is dancing with Melanie, who is dressed as a cocktail waitress among many cocktail waitresses, nurses, and corseted callgirls.

Suddenly, the crowd pushes to the side and I turn to see Yanni and his friends making their entrance. One of his entourage is a man-child with a streaky mane of red hair; he stops to stretch his arms over his head, which displays the glistening, interwoven muscles of his back. Two attractive women in bikinis and sarongs stand on either side of Yanni, their palms against his trim waist. They smell like sex.

A tall black man follows them. Yan points me out and the man staggers over to me, puts his arms around me, grips my backside and begins to sway. For several beats I am too shocked to resist or to take in what he is saying to me. When I regain my wits, I realize that he is an American, and gather that Yanni is in the midst of an orgy that started at Bell's Beach, continued in his van on the ride to Denton, and will be continuing here. As I pull away, the American—presumably Hawk—gives me a play-by-play of what they have all done together so far, which both disturbs and revolts me. He then says that Yanni has told him that I am a fan of his basketball team and of him and am a tantrika who could teach him many things.

He adds, "Yanni passed around some drugs. I don't know what they were."

I put my hands on either side of his face and try to look him in the eyes. "I can take you to the kitchen, give you something to eat, and drink some strong Greek coffee with you. If you like, you can take a class with me. It will be sweet, and loving, and chaste; a good antidote to Yanni's careless profanity."

Hawk chokes out a laugh. "I don't want to stop now. I could go for hours." His erect penis pushes my belly as he whispers in my ear, "I want to do it with you up at the tent."

I pull away, hold him at arm's length and say, "I'm afraid Yanni's been having you on. I don't practice the left-hand path. I don't even have sex. I'm celibate."

Hawk stumbles and jerks his head. "You're really a nun?"

I don't know how to tell him what I am, so I simply nod.

"Oh," Hawk says with a laugh. "Good one. How about that hottie over there in the bunny costume?"

"You mean Yanni's wife?"

"Yeah! She looks ... wow!"

I wriggle away and run out, afraid of being a pawn in Yanni's bizarre party crashing. The night is beginning to feel like a nightmare. I look back and catch a glimpse of Hawk enfolding Melanie in his long arms. I hope that he does not tell her the story of his ride with Yanni the way he told it to me. I hope I can escape before becoming party to Yanni's spite.

When I spot Graeme on the patio, I run at him to tell him what Yanni is up to, and what its consequences must be—but when I am almost face to face with him, he nods sadly as if he has heard my thoughts. I stop in shock and lock eyes with him.

Something happens that is outside the range of my understanding. In the space between my brows, at the place of the third or inner eye, I see a vision that is like a tunnel through the third eyes of all of those present in this place. I see Steve forcing me in bed; Melanie absorbing Yanni's rage in the act of union; Gyorgos taking beatings from school mates; Gyorgos watching Yanni descend into the realm of animals; Yanni enduring a seemingly endless string of failures that culminate in a covert suicide attempt in the swells beyond Bell's Beach; Grandma lying heartbroken on her husband's grave; Hal cut off from his father's love; Judy's heart pierced by Roger's indiscretions; and Ruth struck by Grandma's hard will.

The vision is merciless. It continues through the tunnel of connected minds, boring into secrets and miseries that could break a mind unable to face the fierce grace of perfect memory. The tunnel ends in Graeme's mind. I see his father beating him with a belt, and I see the heart-shattering loss of a paralyzed partner. I realize with amazement that these horrific scenes are now offset with compassion that overrides their pain: Graeme can respond to them as he chooses. It is my mind, now, that is supplying any distress.

The vision shifts from the tunnel to a black starry sky. Graeme's voice says in my mind, "Join us for the class, and bring Andy." At the bottom of the image is a dark pool that is rippled on the surface. Packets of light move outward from the center and expand in shimmering rings of transformation that extend through space and time. Ordinary consciousness exists outside this shared vision in which I feel Graeme and Reggie answering pain with purification. I see now that their class is not only for consorts; it is for all who hurt and would transform it into sweet love to interweave hearts across barriers and voids.

I see that I could not partner Graeme if I wished to; my small equanimity cannot hold such extremes of pain and ecstasy, nor remain resiliently loving and at the same time fully aware of malice. The vision continues, and becomes too much for me. Graeme has already communicated far more than I can receive. I put my fingers over the place between my brows and stumble away, shaking with sorrow and horror.

Before I have regained my wits, I hear Andy's voice ask, "Are you all right, mate?" I turn to see him standing beside the iron lace table, one foot up on a heavy white chair, dressed as a bush guide in tiny shorts and a shirt with pockets. He is cleaning his nails with a huge bush knife.

"No! I'm spinning like a kid on a carnival ride at Luna Park." I take a seat beside him and rub my forehead with my forefinger. "I just saw Hawk, and he told me what Yanni's been up to, which is very distressing, and then I saw Graeme, which was—well—weird. I thought I was ready for all of this, but I'm not. I just want to go home, wherever that is."

"You complaining about the stables, now?" Andy asks acerbically.

I shake my head. I am not equal to rough humor. Not now.

"What's Yan done this time?"

"He started an orgy with his mates, and he's planning to continue it here."

"Crickey. That bludger could cool any hot investor. Anything else?"

"I'm not ready to sit with Graeme, so he wants me to come to the tantra class with you, which must mean that he wants you to win your bet."

"Don't worry. You can count on me."

"What am I counting on you for? I have no idea what I'm doing."

"You can count on him to be your friend," says Lisa's lightly accented voice. I turn to see her approaching with a sweating stubby in each hand. She is petite, with thick silken black hair, a taupe complexion, liquid amber eyes, and swollen breasts that fill the folds of her Hawaiian costume. She holds a cold one out to Andy. "We're making a go of it again, thanks to you."

I start to cry. I can't stop. The prospect of something turning out well is more than I can handle. I stand and hug her tightly. She hugs me back. When she releases me I say with a laugh, "We have to stop hugging like this."

Lisa laughs and says cheekily, "I like it."

"You know, Andy, I think I'm finally wearing the right outfit."

"You look crook, Collo, but you'll come right when you take off that daft costume."

"Good idea. But I should tell Gyorgos about Yan, shouldn't I?"

"Lisa will pay him a little visit. Gyorgos won't be able to stop Yanni now, but he'll want to know."

I reach out and squeeze Andy's hand, and Lisa's. "You're true blue, mates, true blue."

Andy kisses Lisa tenderly, takes my elbow, and says, "Let's take a little stroll."

He leads me on a circuitous route west and then north and east, maintaining silence and pausing now and then to see if we are being followed. I feel as if I'm back in school, this time as both teacher and pupil. I'm content with having learned my lesson for the day, which is that I have untold work to do before I can handle the full spectrum of reality with equanimity, and that I should leave unfolding events to those who can see them clearly—including Andy, who is coming through as a friend in need, a friend indeed.

We round the poplar trees and cut across the pasture to the

hothouse, where I lift the plastic flap and release warm, moist air and the murmur of intimate exchanges. Inside, I see upturned crates holding clusters of candles that reveal a transformed interior. Tarps and cushions cover the ground; the plastic wall between the hothouse and laboratory is gone; and against the far wall stands a low dais mounded with multicolored cushions. Reggie and Graeme are sitting on them facing each other. Graeme is wearing a plain karate robe, and Reggie is in a shiny bra and harem pants. On the laboratory floor and between the raised garden beds, twenty or so partially dressed couples sit in similar fashion, talking quietly as they wait for the class to begin. Between the far garden beds and the north wall, a few couples are wearing nothing at all. To my surprise, Liz and Ronnie are among them, sitting and giggling together as Liz caresses Ronnie's shoulders.

Andy and I go to take our seats on a pile of green pillows near Hal and Dutchy, who are themselves near to Laura and Clive, Louis and Emily, and Rog and Judy. Fortunately, they are all too interested in each other to pay us heed. Andy and I soon find a way to sit facing without touching each other or disturbing our neighbors. We sink into the atmosphere, which is loving and expectant. The energy is low and still, but increasing in intensity.

Almost as soon as we take our seats, Graeme begins speaking in a slow, warm, gravelly voice.

"Welcome. Reg and I have invited you to join us here tonight to share the basics of our sacred sexual practice. As some of you know, my practice comes out of tantric Buddhism, and Reggie's out of a sister tradition from India. For us, the sexual practice supports a continuous practice that affects every moment of our lives and every aspect of our experience. It supports us to know and love each other better; to perceive, penetrate, and dissolve sources of darkness; and to deepen and clarify our conscious union with all sources of life.

"We haven't taught together before, so we'll be sharing the most basic practices and asking how they affect you and your partner. We encourage you to recognize that this time is dedicated to deepening the sacred bond that you already have. Some of you may have viewed your bond as a mystery and allowed it to develop outside your awareness, in the subconscious and unconscious parts of your body. Our aim in sharing our practice is for you to enhance your awareness of the joy and creativity inherent in your bond, and to help you enhance and develop it.

"We also aim for you to be able to use the practices for strength and clarity as well as enjoyment. You'll want to do that from the start, because when you open, you and your partner expose vulnerabilities and reveal and release obstacles. If either of you lacks transparency, the union will be incomplete, and you may lack the skill or strength to transform darkness into light in a way that deepens states of bliss and supports synergy in daily life. While you're here, we can support your practice, but away from us you may go through a trial by fire. Don't be afraid of it; that's the part of the practice that opens and purifies you for sacred union and deepening happiness.

"Your experience today is likely to begin quite joyfully, and to give you a taste of the bliss and freedom that come of a mature practice. But if you've never done silent prayer or meditation, an obstacle may arise early on that may be quite painful or challenging. If you need help or have questions, we invite you to call on us."

Reggie says, "This evening we're going to share a little poetry and a few simple exercises."

Graeme says, "We'll start with Rumi. He was a Sufi poet and religious leader who freed the hearts and minds of his fellow students of Islam from the tyranny of intellectualism. His followers recognized union with a lover as a first step toward union with God."

Reggie continues, "Sufis also practice loving at will. Their poetry can help us to open and purify our hearts. It's ancient, but is just as useful today in offsetting the excess information and disinformation of modern life."

Graeme asks, "Does anyone have a question before we start?"

Hal raises his hand. "I'm Jewish. I don't know anything about Sufism and I don't want to practice it."

"That isn't a problem from our side," Reggie replies. "If you like, you can become familiar with the feeling of a practice and observe its short- and long-term effects, and you and your partner can adapt it to suit your existing faith and practice."

Graeme adds, "When we've started, you can signal us to come and help you sort it."

"Let's start with a simple practice," Reggie says, her voice shifting from supportive to instructive. "I want you to close your eyes and allow the ear of your heart to open to these words."

When Andy closes his eyes, I close mine. I have read some of Reggie's books of Rumi's poetry rendered by Bly, Barks, Cowan, and Harvey, but when Graeme reads, I don't recognize the poems he has chosen. His voice is a resonant bass that vibrates through our bones, and is at once both earthy and ecstatic. It comes from a realm in which physical union is not separate from love, divinity, or metamorphosis.

Reggie says tenderly, "Take turns pouring words of love from your heart into your lover's ears. When it is your turn to listen, let your ears drink in your lover's words."

For a minute, Andy and I remain silent. Then he says, "I thought when you came out to Australia that you'd take Reg away from me. It's been the opposite, and I'm grateful."

My heart fills with sweet sisterhood. I reply, "I count my blessings in your capability, your strength, and your loyalty to your mates and your vocation."

Reggie says to Graeme, and to all of us, "Put your hand on your lover's heart and tell your love without words."

After a bit of awkward fumbling, Andy and I press our palms together. Joy and arousal fill the space around us. I close my eyes and pray. My chest fills with white light that spreads beyond our flesh and joins with the all that no mind can hold alone.

I sit serenely. I feel the warmth of Andy's palms and no more, and I open my eyes to be sure that he, too, is calm and happy. His eyes are closed; I wonder if he is dozing.

Sometime later, Graeme intones another tactile and transcendent rhapsody of untamed love and unbounded exploration. His rich, deep bass interpenetrates words and thoughts and carries his tone of sweet surrender into a sensual experience of divinity. I look at Graeme and see that he has let his robe fall in folds; I also see that Reggie has removed her bra. He is nude, now, and she is nearly so. I look around the room and see that Hal and Dutchy, Laura and Clive, and Louis and Emily are absorbed in each other. I close my eyes and allow my body to abide in the ocean of love that we are creating and sharing. Soon, I feel the powerful erotic currents of intimacy in company. My breathing deepens.

Graeme's voice intones an ecstatic ode with a calm that helps to ground our embodied union, and then Reggie says, "Look through your partner's eyes into the source of joy and love. When the barriers that divide you become transparent, rest in wonder. Embrace your lover and enhance your union with a kiss."

Andy and I smile at each other and then close our eyes and do not kiss. My breathing slows and seems to stop, and ripples of joy play up and down on either side of my spine. Later, when a tingling like a valley of ecstasy begins at my root, intensifies, rises, and fills the cup of my being, I wonder if the atmosphere could carry us away, and whether it is time for Andy and me to go.

I open my eyes. Andy tips his head toward the door. I nod. As we rise and approach the door flap, we hear footsteps running up to the door from outside, and Geoffrey's voice lamenting, "Yanni and his friends are having an orgy in the big tent. They've taken the horses in! One of them could break a leg in that mass of flesh!"

I hear shuffling on the dais, and look to see Reggie putting on her clothes. She says, in a besotted voice that turns steely, "Emily and Laura, find Melanie and Ruth and make sure they take the children upstairs in the big house. Dutchy and Lisa, tell the deejay and guests the party's over. The rest of you, get ready to go with Graeme and me to the south pasture. Can you do that?"

"Is that really necessary?" Graeme asks quietly.

Before Reggie can reply, distant screams break into the dream of tranquil ecstasy that stamped our bodies with a sweet state of surrender. Now, a state of alarm turns the air of the hothouse thick and phantasmagoric, so that it seems that we are moving through deep waters and seeing through lenses that darken and distort their shadowy depths.

Andy and I rush outside and run after Geoff, toward the south pasture; we soon overtake him. I look back and see that the others are following closely. I fall behind Andy, who runs nimbly along the stony path that leads due south across the east pasture to the practice track. I come fully awake to the cold night, realizing that we are unprepared for whatever trouble lies ahead, and that we may have no idea how to meet it or to mend it.

Soon, all of my attention is focused on my footing. Unlike the familiar path to the hothouse, which I can walk in the dark or half-asleep, this one is grassy, rocky, and uneven. I worry that one of us may sprain an ankle on a stone, leave a patch of skin on a fence rail or a thorny shrub, or trip and fall in a pile of sheep scat—but Andy guides us well. We are all fortunate that Yanni's provocation led Andy to the group in the hothouse. I lift the skirts of my habit and follow his steps across the pasture, through the bush-lined brook where the shy platypus may be hiding in terror as our feet pound by, and up the south hilltop where we pause to take in a panorama of brutal confusion.

The tent and track lights are on, spotlighting the big white canvas tent on our left as well as the finish line of the practice track on our right. A dynamic knot of nude men first appears to be engaged in a footy play on the cloddy earth of the practice track; a second look reveals that they are fighting fitfully with sticks and rocks. The back of the tent is swaying as if a crew inside is taking it down, but its irregular bulge and the silhouettes playing on its wall show that a horse is rearing against the back wall, and that scattered partygoers are attempting to run or crawl away from the animal's sharp hooves. We hear a neigh of terror, shrill screams, and the collapse of metal furniture. A sheep darts out of and away from the tent toward the darkness of the eastern bush. We see scattered figures lying here and there on the ground in its path and realize that they are not resting; they are injured. It is like a picture of Pagan sex painted by an angry Christian priest, a lusty scene of rapine violation imprinting bodies with self-perpetuating patterns of pain and strife and suffering.

"What should we do?" I ask Andy.

"I don't know. We don't want to provoke them."

As we stand there confused, a clot of figures rushes from the eastern bush to the tent. We hear shouts of rage and see that one of the figures is carrying a burning stick. In seconds, smoke begins to rise from the far corner of the tent; a red glow illuminates the clot of figures and the treetops that rise above them like empty watchtowers. As the group from the hothouse gathers around us, we all stand transfixed by the dancing fire of Shiva-destruction. I tear my eyes away and see Graeme holding Reg, who appears distracted. Both are crying.

Andy moves first; we all follow him to the front of the tent, which is wide open to the night. Andy shouts, "Gerry, drop that stick or I'll tell your father where you've been! Ken! Andrew! Davey! Skip! Allan!"

The figures from the eastern bush look up at him like a band of stags and then rush back and disappear into the trees. The figure with the burning stick drops it and follows them, as do several of the nude men who were fighting on the track.

Emily shouts fearfully from behind us, "Get out of that tent, you bloody idiots!"

Naked figures are already running or staggering out onto the practice track. Some turn and run toward the big house, while others limp away to sit or lie down on the track. A horse gallops out between them and disappears due south in the direction of the bluff that overlooks the city lights.

Louis calls out desperately, "Come smother the flames!"

Louis organizes a group to pull on the tent ropes on the bush side of the tent; he and Andy and I run to the opposite side to untie and release the ropes. With a great heave, the others pull on the swaying tent. The poles tilt. The canvas billows, momentarily fanning the flames; then it topples onto the flames and smothers them. Smoke fans out from under the tent, stinging eyes and choking lungs. Roger opens his fly and pisses on the embers; others quickly do the same. The fire is soon quenched.

"People are trapped inside!" Emily shouts.

The tent bulges irregularly. A muffled cry of anguish rises from the far corner, followed by an animal scream of alarm from the collapsed front. We hear coughing, and the sounds of metal chairs and tables sliding and colliding. Weak voices rise from the center.

Andy grabs a fold of canvas in the fallen roof of the tent near the far corner and holds it up; he grips his bush knife, stabs the fabric, and pulls the knife against it until a slit opens. He steps up on the lumpy canvas and cuts along the weft of the fabric until he has extended the gash by several feet, and then several yards. Rog and Louis, and then Judy and Dutchy, rush awkwardly up the bumpy canvas, grab the edges on either side of the tear, and pull until the old fabric gives way and opens a gash that extends all the way from one side to the other.

As I watch, I seem to see the surface of the earth open and release curses past and present. Bodies emerge like Loki's children from the body of the demon Angerboda. A horse struggles to its feet from under a torn bit of canvas; seeing its wild eyes and sharp hooves, we scatter to make way. The animal makes a decision and bolts west, trailing a garland of ripped crepe paper; a scream rises from beneath its hooves. Then Yanni himself rises from the folds of the tent, his foreskin stuck to the hair inside his left thigh, his scalp bleeding profusely down his back. He sways unsteadily; his chiseled features contort hideously and he screams in the direction of the eastern bush, "I'll bugger you for this!"

"You're going to hell!" shouts a high voice from the bush. "They should take your kid away!"

Another voice shouts, "You're all Sodomites! You'll all burn for eternity!"

"*Going* to hell?" Reg counters tensely, her voice breaking. "Isn't this it?"

Yanni screams, "This is private property! We can shag any way we please!"

Yanni presses his hand to his scalp as several bodies wriggle free of the tent. One rushes toward the path to the big stone house. A jagged ring of onlookers gathers, crying or gaping in shock at the smoldering tent. We catch a glimpse of glistening flesh squirming on the tent floor under a table. Stepping carefully over the lumpy canvas, I reach the table and help a young, naked woman out of the tent. She grabs my arm and begins rambling about the boys who came from the bush to peep into the tent and how one came inside to have sex with her but pulled out and ran when he saw his mates.

"Why did he run away from me? Why?" she asks plaintively.

I put my arms around her and hold her as she cries. When she has become calmer, I ask, "Was a black American in there with you?"

She doesn't reply.

"You need to cover up," I say, looking around for the tough but maternal Laura. When I find her in the outer circle of distraught faces, I put my arm around the girl, walk her to Laura, and ask, "Do you have any extra clothes for this girl?"

Laura nods, puts her arm around the girl, and leads her gently but firmly toward the south guest yurt. I join several others who are pulling debris from the tent and searching it for any stragglers who may still be trapped inside. As Rog, Louis, and Judy work systematically through the wreckage, I see Andy kneeling on the practice track beside a young man with a bloody gash in his knee. Seeing me, he says, "Collo, I need strips of cloth. Can you rip up that witch costume?" As I struggle with the old black fabric, he shouts, "Hoy, Hal!"

"Ay?" Hal calls back.

"Call a general surgeon and have him meet us at the nearest emergency ward! When you've done that, get transport and a first aid kit down here."

As I pull off my cowl and bite on the cloth to tear away strips from its edge, I see Hal procure a mobile phone from Louis and take charge of the transport of the injured. I fetch Andy's knife and cut strips from my costume that he uses to dress the young man's wound. When he is satisfied, he tells the man to lie still for now and motions me to follow him to another man who is lying nearby. All around us, women in nurse costumes are tending to injured men in fancy dress. It is like the set of a action film invaded by the cast of a porn movie.

Clive retrieves a first aid kit from his vehicle. Emily and two other horse owners drive their trucks to the track; they and Dutchy and several others transport the injured who need no first aid or who have been bandaged, some of whom must be carried. Hal directs them to a local surgeon's office.

"This is all on you, Pappas, you arsehole!" a voice screams from the circle gathered around the tent. I look and see that the redheaded man with the streaky mane is enraged at Yanni. He and his mates have stopped on the path to the house in order to turn back and make rude hand gestures at Yanni. The circle of onlookers breaks up as those who can walk head for the path. I call after a small group of angry women, "Did you see a black American?"

One pauses and calls back to me, "He left with Melanie."

Soon, our friends have finished folding the tent, setting aside the articles that were inside it, and escorting away stragglers who are in shock but are able to leave. Then only Andy and I and several injured boys remain at the desolated site. I am shuddering. After the bath of love in the hothouse, the misery on the field feels like a cold Buddhist hell.

"I think there are only six."

"One bloke's lying in the dark over that way," Andy says, pointing east.

"I didn't see him."

"We'd better have a look."

We find a young man unconscious on the turf near the far end of the track. As we lift him, cradling his head and neck and shifting him onto a piece of canvas, I find that I am no longer as strong as I was. I do what I can to help Andy lift the man's dead weight and carry him at a fast pace toward the place where we expect the next vehicle to arrive.

"Thank God," I say as a truck rolls down the gravel track from the new stables. "Almost there."

Rog, Louis, and Clive converge on the spot. Andy directs them to help find and carry the injured, while Geoffrey arrives and directs me to help him find the skittish horses who are wandering or waiting at the edge of the southern bush. I trade with Louis, who knows race horses and will be better able to aid

Geoffrey. When we have filled the truck, it goes rolling gently but quickly up the hill; Andy and I remain at the scene to make a final sweep of the tent and the track.

"That's it, then. Let's go up," Andy says conclusively as he turns out the spotlights. "You okay?"

"Holding steady. You?"

"Christ!" he says. "Bloody hell!"

"I didn't get a chance to thank you for sitting with me." I take Andy's hand and clasp it. "We'll all be fine. Once we recover."

"This is the end. This is the bloody end of all of it. I reckon my job's finished."

"No, Reg will figure it out. We three will. You can count on us."

Andy snorts, but then heaves a big sigh. His body relaxes; he has been in shock. Once he releases me with a rough squeeze, we turn and walk up toward the big stone house. As we approach, we see Reggie talking with Yanni at the hedge near the front entry. She is saying sadly but sternly, "Yan, I know you're suffering, but your self-pity is deadly and you're the only one who can change it."

A bandage has stopped Yanni's bleeding. He appears soberer than he was, but sounds whiny and resentful. "Always so sodding self-righteous!"

"Do you really think you can offend me with harsh speech after defiling Denton Stables in the name of everything I hold sacred?" Yanni opens his mouth to retort, but only shakes his head in contempt. Reggie continues, "You've chosen destruction over creation, death over life. I'm done with you."

"Piss off."

"You'll have to leave. Gyorgos will look after baby Niko and Melanie. From now on, you'll have to find your own way. We can't help you."

"I don't need you! I don't need anyone."

"You'll be glad, then, won't you?" Reggie says perfunctorily as she turns away.

12

Parlay

While Yanni hangs back as if reluctant to enter the house, we hear a short wail of a siren and see a lone police car rolling up the drive. Yanni disappears around the back of the house. The car parks at the front steps, and an elderly officer emerges. His head is round and bald; his features and build are bulbous. He goes straight inside. Andy and I catch him up in the kitchen, where Reggie is standing with her mother. They are talking in low, somber voices. The officer interrupts them with criticisms of the changes that Gyorgos has made to the kitchen. He introduces himself as Detective Trask and puts the kettle on. Reggie looks at Andy and me; we share a shrug and a puzzled look.

We all take seats at the huge butcher-block table as Detective Trask explains that he was the only detective on duty when a consultant called from the hospital to report yet another Cup party gone wrong. He tells us that he will begin his investigation once he has had his tea. Yanni, who has thrown on some work clothes that were hanging on a peg near the kitchen garden, enters the back way, sits on a stool and crosses his arms with a truculent frown.

Andy sets his arms on the table, rests his head on his arms, and closes his eyes. My mind scatters; Reggie brings me back by asking me to fetch Gyorgos. I take a deep breath and obey, hoping that he will not explode. I creep up the stairs and knock reluctantly on the door of the big blue room. I hear Ruth's voice, but can't make out her words.

I open the door a crack and say, "Gyorgos, the police are here, and Reggie wants you to come down."

After a pause, Gyorgos swears in Greek, thumps around the room, and bursts out of the door pulling a black robe over pink silk pajamas.

Ruth calls out, "Colette! Has anyone seen Melanie? We couldn't find her or baby Niko."

"She left with Hawk."

"Hawk?"

"He's the guy Yanni said he invited for me. He, um, got caught in the chaos."

"Wait a minute."

Ruth emerges in her robe. We return to the kitchen and take seats at the table. The detective finishes his tea and dutifully questions us about the evening's events. I know almost nothing of police work, but find it odd that he doesn't separate the witnesses or take notes, and assume that it means that he will not be taking anyone away to jail.

When each of us has told the story as we know it, and Gyorgos' face has gone from flushed to sickly green, Detective Trask concludes, "I don't think anyone'll be pressing charges. They're all kids, and most will have been traumatized by the sexual nature of the situation. There's no need for the law to make it worse, or to break your grandmother's heart. She's always been so good to me."

He sighs and looks into his empty cup. "We needn't disturb

her now. I'll go have a talk with the elders next door. One of you had better come along and start mending fences. I don't have to tell you how they'll feel about what their boys saw here."

"And I don't have to tell you how I feel about their trespassing, or their attempted murder of Yanni and his friends," Gyorgos says sharply, "or that my barrister could find a way to put them all away for a long time."

"It's a good thing we take pride in our community relations, Gyorgos, and that we don't want to make a name for ourselves with this case. That saves me filling the gaol with your lot."

"Thank you, officer," Reggie says. "We're grateful for your wisdom and experience."

"It's hard to say how the press would view the Brethren," Gyorgos seethes stubbornly. "They don't make it easy on young people who don't belong. Yanni's very popular up here, and I'm sure a lot of people would be glad to speak on his behalf."

"Ah, don't get up yourself, you overblown tucker tosser. Yanni's a lost cause, and everyone in the district knows it and wants him gone."

Reggie says evenly. "Would you like me or Gyorgos to go with you?"

"The conciliatory one, or the angry one?" Trask frowns thoughtfully. "I'll take the angry one, thanks. That'll make a matched set. And keep Yanni out of sight, will you, luv? He's already shown everyone in Port Phillip heaps more than they wanted to see."

Detective Trask stands and leans forward on his hands, elbows straight. He says to Anne, "Good bye, luv."

Once Detective Trask has left, the anger that was simmering in Gyorgos erupts. He shouts at Yanni, "You could at least try to look sorry!" And then he hurries after the detective.

"How are the injured?" Reg asks Andy.

"One was out cold, one may need a new knee, a few needed sewing up, and there may have been a few broken bones and concussions—but I reckon they'll all recover."

We drink tea in near silence until Gyorgos returns. He is grim but sanguine. He has met with two elders of the Plymouth Brethren who expressed upset and criticism of both sides, and who quickly agreed to handle the aftermath without legal action. Gyorgos thanks us for tending the wounded. I notice with a shock that Yanni has already recovered his usual magnetism. I am astonished that the night has done nothing to mar his beauty, and realize with a jolt that this night may have followed the usual pattern of his life. Reg has also recovered much of her usual composure.

Ruth says to Reg, with barely controlled anger and distress, "I blame you for putting ideas into their heads! You and Yan will have to leave."

I say, "Yan is obviously a hazard and Reg's talents as a wine-maker are wasted here. And you—who can't tell sacred sex from profane sex—and Yan—for whom nothing is sacred—even vilify her for her finest accomplishments as a human being! Plus, Andy and I want nothing more to do with a family that would create this kind of havoc and then blame it on her."

"You're not even family!" Ruth declares.

"She's done a lot more for The Inn than you have," Anne observes. "But I'd like to hear what Reg has to say."

As Reg inhales to speak, Gyorgos interjects, with a flourish of his robe, "Hedonists and end-times cultists deserve each other!"

As she attempts to speak again, Yanni says as if hoping to be contradicted, "It's my fault."

"You'll have to leave," Ruth says sharply. "And Melanie has to keep your child away from you!"

"Before you get carried away managing Denton," Anne says peremptorily to Ruth, "you should know that Grandma will be leaving everything to Reggie."

After a stunned silence, Gyorgos, who appears incensed, sputters, "She brought us here and now she's throwing us out? Outrageous!"

"No," Anne says, "She believes that Reg—having no children—will be the least partial."

Reggie says with a sigh, "She has a lot of respect for you, Gyorgos, and knows that I lack your golden touch, and fears that I'll fail to earn an income."

"What do you think, Mum?" Yanni asks with an eerie tone of innocence.

"I think you'd all but left Melanie and that there was no need for any of this to have occurred and you should have seen that."

"But the will, Mum. What do you think Grandma means by it?"

"I think she knows that Reggie will take care of all of us. Gyorgos' primary obligation is to Ruth and the children. And you have no prospects."

"You told her to do it, didn't you, Mum?" Yanni asks with a frown.

"Nobody tells Grandma to do anything, Yanni, and you know it. I gave her advice when she needed it, and she usually took it, but none was needed in this case. I'm too old to manage Denton, and Dad left you all well provided for—too well, in your case. You're spoilt and I'm ashamed of you."

"Look, Gyorgos," Reggie says, "whatever the legalities, I want you and your family to live here and develop The Inn. I think we all know that I'll have to go, too, for a decade at least."

Ruth's eyes gleam hopefully. I imagine Grandma striking Ruth with her cane.

"Why should you?" Gyorgos says, more upset by Reggie's generosity than by Grandma's caprice. I can see from Ruth's face that Gyorgos' vision of family business has more to do with Reggie than with Ruth. For him, the only thing worse than life with Yanni is life without Reggie. He calms himself and then says tensely, "Ruth's upset. We're all upset! Imagine if the tent had burned! No one blames you for Yanni's idiocy."

"Gyorgos, I love you of course, all of you, but you can thrive with a conventional wine list, and I'm ready to move on. And while I don't believe in taking offense, I don't believe in asking for it either. I want to live with Graeme and love him openly without the burden of secrecy," Reggie's voice catches, "and without anyone coming between us or cursing us with contempt. I want to work at one of the old wineries in the Yarra, and already asked the present owner of one of them, George Wheeler, for a position."

Andy and I look at each other open-mouthed.

Gyorgos replies, "Victoria Regina, we've always supported you, as you've supported us."

"I know. And I will continue to support you. Look, you must see that we need a family strategy to cope with this scandal. If Yan and I leave, you and Geoffrey can put the blame on us and save The Inn. If all goes well, we can return later."

Ruth holds her tongue. I hold my breath.

"It's time we went to bed," Anne says sternly. She stands and pushes her chair under the table with a loud scrape. "We can sort ourselves in the morning."

"Good night, Mum," Reggie says, rising to give her mother a tight hug. "Thanks for taking all of this so well."

When Anne is gone, Reggie gestures to Andy and the three of us leave the house and cross the drive. Fifty yards to the south, we spot two strange figures moving slowly, muttering and moving their arms. A chill goes up my back. At first, I think they are visions; then I see that they are Aboriginal men in white paint. "Reggie! Who are they?"

Reggie stops, looks at them, and whispers, "I think Graeme called them to come and help mend the damage to the land. We should move on, let them work."

Epilogue

Reggie moves swiftly down toward the stables; Andy and I follow to the courtyard and into her room. Reg plops down on her bed, Andy on the floor, and I on her desk chair.

She begins, "I just want to thank you for the amazing work that you did here, and to apologize for what happened today."

"It wasn't your lookout. It was Yan's. The—" Andy is seething now that he is reminded of all that happened, but stops short of speaking ill of Reg's family.

"I hope you don't mind what I said to Ruth," I say.

"Ah, look, I try to avoid polarization and oppositional thinking, but my family's too much for me sometimes. I'm chuffed that you spoke for me."

"Why didn't you clue us in about Wheeler's place?"

"Graeme saw trouble ahead. I hoped that Yan would go back to his surfing mates satisfied with a little bullying, and leave us in peace with Grandma, but he got high and let himself go."

"When exactly did you apply for this job?" Andy persists.

"I didn't, exactly. I called him to explore the possibility of acquiring a vineyard, and he proposed that I come to work for him as managing oenologist. He's a difficult man, a bit of a yob. His manager and his oenologist walked off the job. He realized that with my skills I could do both. I'd like to give it a go."

"So we're not sure?" I ask.

"Not about that job. But I'm sure that I'm with you in moving toward forming a community that runs a winery, a restaurant, and a retreat center. We have the skills, and while Georgie's creativity may have sparked us, I have no doubt that the three of us can create a group mind and a spirit child—in our case, a center that would make the world a better place."

"With the help of Lisa and Graeme," Andy says.

"Right-o. Graeme could do bodywork, and I'd like Lisa to do our publicity. When she's ready."

"She's got some experience in that area. I reckon she'd like that," Andy muses.

"A new beginning," I say cheekily. "That's what I came here for."

"Do you want to do more training? Leaving will cut off your apprenticeship; there may not be that much work for you at the winery, and we haven't addressed the problem of your citizenship."

"One thing at a time. If we hold the vision of community, I can look out for opportunities and find a way forward."

"We'll come right," Andy says.

"I love you both. Thanks for staying with me."

"What are mates for?"

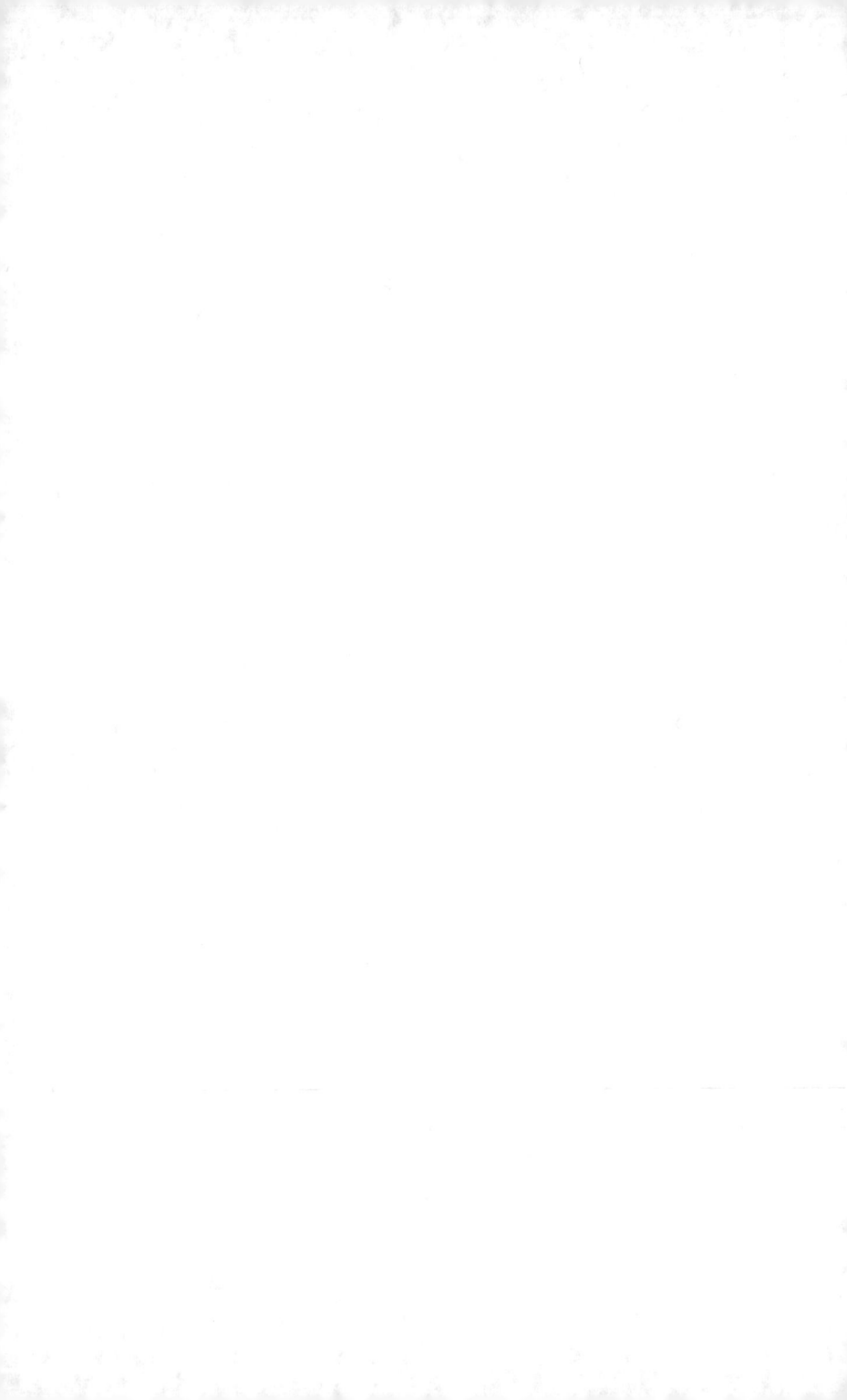

Acknowledgments

The city of Melbourne, Australia, where I lived for two years, inspired the characters, settings, and creativity that shaped this book. I owe a deep debt of gratitude to that city and its state and country, and to the people who shared them with us. A special thanks to hosts Dr. Paul and Mrs. Vivien Zimmet and to Drs. Barb Robertson and Dawn Dewitt. Thank you also to Shiatsu Australia, the Tara Institute, and the Australian medical system for treating me humanely and showing me a contrasting set of strengths and limitations.

For the strengths of culture that revitalized my thinking, I thank the communities of St. Kilda Park Primary and St. Michael's Grammar Schools and the summer holiday programs on Phillip Island. Love and gratitude especially to Principal Sue Knight and parents Chris McAuliffe, Stephanie Holt, Nancy Otis, and Larry Stillman. Through these parents, I found the Victorian Writer's Centre and the Melbourne Arts Centre and its local, national, and international exhibits and performances. All of this—and the programs of the Art Institute of Chicago—fed the character Colette. The beauties and unique features of country Victoria—Hanging Rock, the Yarra Valley, and the Cathedral Range especially—likewise nourished the fictionalized landscape of this part of the Fertility Series saga.

The Acadian aspect of Colette owes a debt to the Midwestern folk music scene and to writer Irène Landry as well as Quebec City's Musée de l'Amérique francophone.

Last and not least, I am grateful to the Southern Oregon team that made this book beautiful. The appearance is due to the professional competence and creativity of cover artist Bruce Bayard and book designer Chris Molé. The readability is due mainly to coach Chansonette Buck and editors Deidre Krupp, Deborah Mokma, and Ann DiSalvo.

Such writing ability as I am developing, I owe first to my father, who taught me reading and writing at a young age. I am also grateful to editor friends Eva Silverfine and Stephanie Holt for their talent and skill in verbal expression, and to writing teachers: Andrea Goldsmith of the Victorian Writer's Centre and Wendy Call of Hugo House. They kindly put up with an unusual and neurotoxic student, trusting that their wisdom would not go to waste.

Thank you also to my book development and beta readers, especially: Jan Agosti, Anna Barón, Jessica Bondy, Cynthia Bradley, Julie Clayton, Stephanie Holt, Christopher Howell, Joel Mason, Sara Myers Wade, Berta Nicol-Blades, and Dana Smaller. Special thanks to Jan, Anna, Julie, and Stephanie for their kindness in dark times.

About the Author

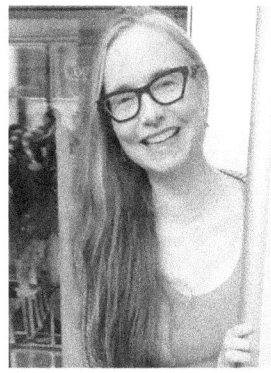

Beth Alderman, MD, MPH earned her AB and MD degrees from the University of Chicago and her MPH from the University of Washington. After Board Certification in Preventive Medicine and Public Health, she took a faculty position in the University of Colorado Medical School Department of Preventive Medicine, Biometrics, and Medical Informatics, where she did population-based epidemiological studies of adverse reproductive outcomes and methodological studies in clinical epidemiology. In her next faculty position at the University of Washington School of Public Health, she focused on risk factors for birth defects.

In 1996, she fell ill with the mysterious new plague and was given the provisional diagnosis "chronic fatigue syndrome". She has spent her time since studying her own case and pondering the reasons that her beloved profession failed her so completely. Fortunately, she discovered her cure, which may be of use to others suffering from one or more of the emerging epidemics affecting humans, their habitats, and life on earth.

For more about and from the author, see the following websites:

BethAldermanMD.com	*Free Information for all readers*
DoctorsOfLife.com	*For care and cure of all lives as one*
LivingFutureBooks.com	*Publishing Website*
LivingFutureCourses.com	*Educational Website with Free and advanced Courses*

Look for author's books on Amazon.com

Other Books by
Beth Alderman

Medical Phenomenology:
Chronic Ambient Poisoning

ISBN: 978-1-7332849-2-9

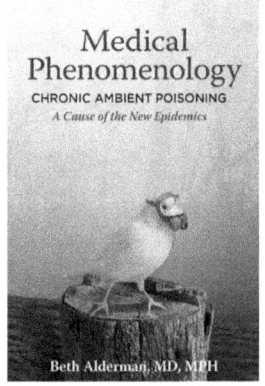

One day in December of 1996, the author (a physician, medical detective, and academic epidemiologist) developed disabling brain fog following on a decade-long descent into a painful, pervasive, and unprecedented chronic illness. Having done population-based studies to research the causes of birth defects, and having thus encountered the limitations of modern methods, she had inadvertently prepared to investigate the causes of her illness—which was given the provisional and uninformative label of "chronic fatigue."

The author began a delineation of the natural history of her condition using the methods of: doctors Hippocrates, Maimonides and Oliver Sacks; the "radical empiricism" used by Dr. William James; and the phenomenology introduced by Teilhard de Chardin and Merleau-Ponty. After a fifteen-year search, she found a doctor of integrative medicine whose elimination diet relieved her brain fog, which enabled her to complete a self-study and to construct an actionable new diagnosis: chronic ambient poisoning. Unseen by doctors and obscured by medical dogma and a myriad of false diagnoses, chronic ambient poisoning defies late modern, fragmented, accuracy-challenged medical research methods and delivery systems. It also reveals that human-caused habitat injuries that afflict birds, bees, and other species are affecting humans while driving evolved life toward extinction in the way of an asteroid strike. To ignore this diagnosis is to ignore the dangers to all lives posed by maladaptive modern lifeways.

The Evolve Fertility Series

BOOK 1
Melissa's Match: *Great Society*
ISBN: 978-1-7321110-1-1

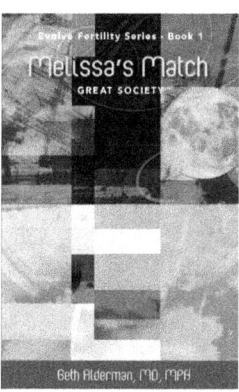

It's the early 1970s. Melissa and her friends begin their first year of college in the inner city of Chicago at a time when post-assassination riots, Great Society scholarship programs, and veterans returning from Vietnam create a sometimes explosive confluence of urban and rural, rich and poor, white and black, educated and uneducated. Coming of age in a violent, unjust, and yet hopeful time, they struggle to reconcile their hopes and opportunities with the shadows of war and the destructive clashes of senescing and emerging systems of care and cure of life on earth.

BOOK 2
Connie's Conception: *Awareness of Peril*
ISBN: 978-1-7321110-0-4

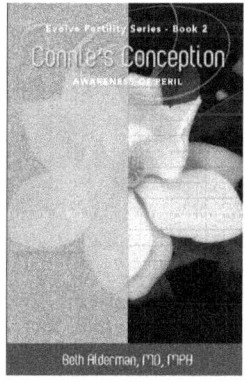

It's the late 1980s, and Connie Martin, a doctor working for the Epidemiology Intelligence Service of the CDC, is called to Colorado to investigate an alarming outbreak of birth defects. Born illegitimate in the San Luis Valley as Consuela Martín, a name known only to close friends and to her beloved gamer and programmer husband, she arrives as an unknown. Joined by environmental activists who suspect the state's Superfund sites and by doctors and parents who fear for its children, Connie attempts to discover the link between habitat destruction and damage to innocents.

BOOK 3
Melissa's Malady: *End of Modernity*
ISBN: 978-1-7321110-2-8

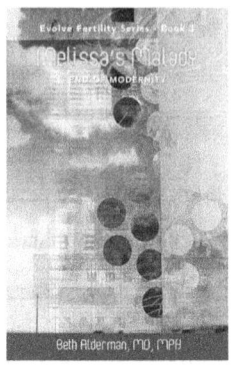

IIt is almost the year of the millennium, and Melissa meets her college friends Sarah and Doug and her first and only true love John for a reunion in Hyde Park. All four are in the midst of their careers. All struggle with the compromises that have marred their happiness. All wish to change the world, each in a different way. Sarah has left her government job for a new life as a yoga teacher. Doug is helping to birth a new value-based economy. John is a successful academic doctor. Melissa is ailing. They unite to turn John's success as a researcher to the cure of Melissa's mysterious chronic illness. What they find will change their lives and their imperiled world.

BOOK 4
Colette's Creativity: *Sacred and Profane*
ISBN: 978-1-7321110-3-5

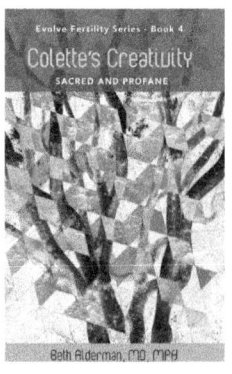

Colette, Melissa's childhood friend, abandons her marriage and home in Maine and flies to Melbourne. There she is taken in by her friend Reggie, who seems to know the secret of joy. Colette joins in the lives of striking individuals who lead her to view sexuality as a manifestation of the sacred. As she leaves behind the wounds caused by profane sexuality, she and her new friends clash with members of Reggie's family who force them to flee and to begin again.

BOOK 5
Colette's Community: *Thirds*
ISBN: 978-1-7321110-4-2

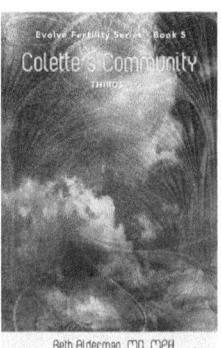

Soon after Colette and her friends find a new home, an old boyfriend of Melissa's who is sojourning in Australia calls and expresses his desire to visit. Colette plans to use the visit as a chance to develop a job for herself; he plans to check up on Colette for Melissa. As they get to know each other, they see that despite differences in religion, origin, and experience, they are on very similar spiritual paths. When it is time for Randall to go home, Colette joins him in Chicago. When he becomes caught up in his old life, however, she returns to Australia to pursue her dream of giving birth to a sacred community.

Chronic Illness Owner's Manuals

Regenerate Your Life: Chronic Illness as a Springboard for Creating Your Best Life

ISBN: 978-1-7321110-8-0 (VOL. 1)
ISBN: 978-1-7321110-9-7 (VOL. 2)

The *Chronic Illness Owner's Manual* series is for patients with chronic illness, and for the people who care for them. Suitable for individual or small group use, it offers a comprehensive, systematic, step-by-step approach to engaging modern medical systems, and to healing from the inside out.

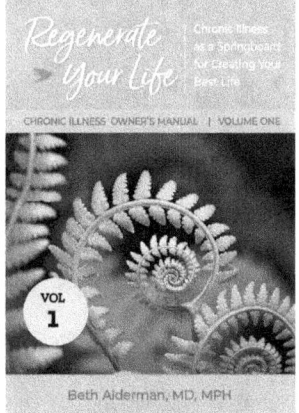

The books comprise anecdotes, exercises, and quotes that address recovery through seven aspects of the body: awareness, understanding, perceptions, sensations, energy, flesh, and interbeing. The frames, constructs, patterns, and processes employed by the series are drawn from traditions of medicine, field biology, theology, and psychology from around the globe. Their synthesis offers an emerging, sustainable, eco-centric, eco-contextual, and customizable approach to creating a new and better life that regenerates your unique meaning, purpose, and vision of abundant life. The *Chronic Illness Owner's Manual* series complements care and cure courses available online at www. LivingFutureCourses.com.

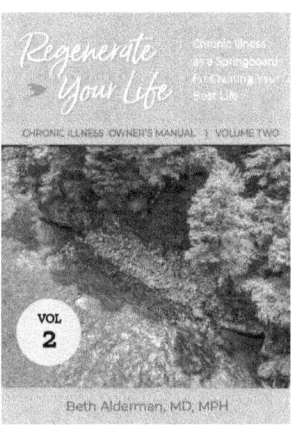

The Evolve Restoration Series
Sequel to the Evolve Fertility Series

BOOK 1
Pilgrim Minds: *After the War on Life*
ISBN: 978-1-7321110-5-9

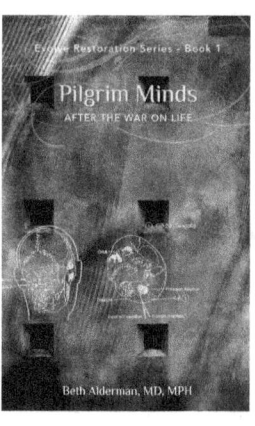

Melissa's deathbed request catapults her son Aaron on a journey from her family's Mississippian clinic to the Salish Sea to claim a mysterious legacy. Meeting his niece Rafa en route, he continues overland with her, and uncle and niece come to know and depend on each other. On arriving at the Saltspring Island Research Center (SIRC), Sarah, now the keeper of the center's narratives, confesses that Aaron's legacy is a task: to apply his mother's philosophy to SIRC's lifeways in order to revitalize it.

While he had been immersed in his mother's medical philosophy, SIRC had used many of her ideas to found a fertility school. SIRC's encroaching apathy persuaded Sarah that they missed one or more essential lifeways, and hopes that Aaron may be able to pinpoint and provide them. Taken by surprise, but ready to step up, Aaron immerses himself in the community, and Rafa undergoes SIRC's initiation process. Uncle and niece come to love Cascadia and to relish local, burgeoning patterns of innovation. Both choose to stay at SIRC, an agentic community that is doing much to restore evolution and its living future.

BOOK 2
Aaron's Legacy: *The Body of Life*
ISBN: 978-1-7321110-6-6

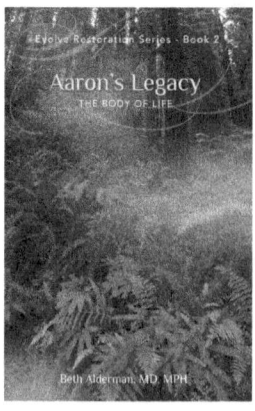

Having come to know the community, Aaron receives his legacy as a series of enactments of SIRC's history. The surviving members of his mother's old friendship group—Sarah, Doug, and John—join the audience and performers in processing and adapting their shared narrative. In the intervals between enactments, Rafa undergoes initiation while Aaron explores the composer, an instrument that enables a player to evoke memories with images and to express the player's responses as sound scapes. As Aaron shares his with Rafa, Sarah and others, John shares memories of Melissa, and seems to receive a new message from her.

As the community adapts to changes in its meaning and purpose, Rafa and Aaron each finds a first consort and draws inspiration from local knowledge keepers and change agents residing at SIRC, the nearby Monastery of Origins and Endings, or in Victoria or Vancouver. Aaron's health, damaged by his travel through a poison barren, deteriorates. With his death, his consort Parvati shares their legacy in the form of patterns of action that may remove roadblocks to continuous adaptation and renewal.

BOOK 3
The Kindred's Rebirth: *Rough Seas and Far Lands*

ISBN: 978-1-7332849-3-6

A decade later in Australia, Parvati and Björn give up on effecting meaningful restoration there. Dirk, while on his annual circuit of the north, arrives in Jokkmokk for the annual Sámi gathering to learn that SIRC is in crisis. Rafa, who is crossing the South Pacific on her two year global clinic circuit, hears strange news: the Fertility School, which was winding down, closed without notice. She realizes that her work, too, is drawing to a close as her clinics adapt to localism and begin to diverge.

All three travelers feel a strong homing urge and hatch a plan to converge in Scandinavia with the remnant of the SIRC community. En route, Parvati adopts a grandchild, Jacki, who helps Björn to recover from a disorder of interbeing. Many new consort pairs join the kindred and revive it by helping to form a next community, SIRC-Umea, and to organize and maintain residential restoration communities in the Baltic and North Sea bioregions, and to recover from the painful loss of the original community.

BOOK 4

Jacki's Vision: *The Green Line*

ISBN: 978-1-7332849-4-3

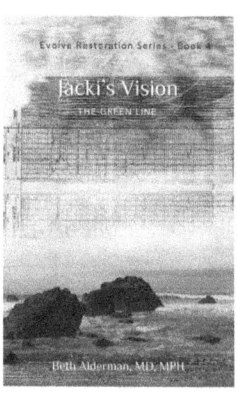

When Jacki turns sixteen, she begins her transition to adulthood by venturing into larger worlds of knowledge and adaptation to gain skills. During her first clinic circuit in the Baltic, she finds that her coming of age is coinciding with her kindred's restiveness. As she embraces and contemplates her future, a vision takes hold of her. She proposes a Green Line restoration project in Tasmania to reconcile a time debt created by the Black Line genocide, and to prepare her for organizing bioregional restoration projects. Her kindred and their networks embrace the project, expand it, and multiply its potential effects.

As the Green Line Corps prepares to depart en masse for Tasmania, Jacki meets a young stranger, Mirek, whose experience of the world—whose very umwelt—contrasts with her own. Later, in Tasmania, she gains a consort, Izaak, and a sister friend, Lally, both of whom winnow her possible futures. Together, the many thousands of Green Line participants develop a restoration ethos and synchronize living processes for restoring habitats—with their restorers. Jacki and her new peers are among the first to return to the original SIRC campus, near which many former kindred members have settled, and to which many others are about to return.

BOOK 5

Mel's Motherhood: *A Place in the Living World*

ISBN: 978-1-7332849-5-0

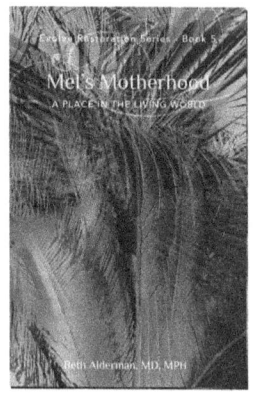

Mel and JJ—children of the Three Mammas—await the advance boat from Tasmania at the Cascadian Monastery of Origins and Endings. Mel, who is pregnant, and JJ, who fared poorly while he was away, finished their initiation projects and are keen to see Jacki and to meet the new kindred members. In the course of a joyful reunion, Mel and JJ learn that Jacki and Lally are also pregnant.

As this next generation of adults chooses ways to express fertility and defines new vocations, the reconstituting kindred celebrates new human lives, integrates with local communities, and processes hitherto hidden threads of SIRC's history with the aid of DNA fathers who participate. The complex, complementary communities adapt to continuous learning via phenomenology, and to continuous adaptation of systems for care and cure of evolved life.

Meaningful Retirement: *Become a Life Care Provider*

ISBN: 978-1-7332849-0-5

Meaningful Retirement is a self-guided monthly course in four seasons that can aid people like you who are exiting modern employment or withdrawing from the modern death economy. In it you will find a toolbox for transition to a vocation of life care, and thus begin to mature into a wise elder able to lead and mentor those who follow you. These seasons include:

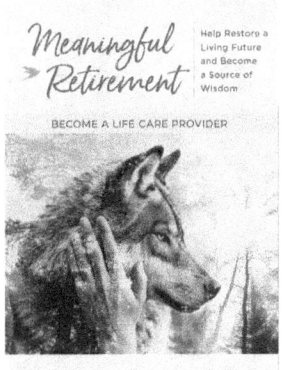

Beth Alderman, MD, MPH

- **A Summer Breather**
- **A Fall for Reflection**
- **A Winter to Reclaim Your Personal Narrative**
- **A Spring for Revolutionizing Your Lifetime Learning**

As you transition to the role of provider of life care, you may choose to co-found emotionally and spiritually astute communities where you can mentor your juniors, who face the imminent and daunting task of passing through wrenching psycho-social change while arresting and reversing the accelerating human-caused Sixth Extinction. That threat to evolved life represents a unique crucible for transforming modern lifeways into ones that enable humans to choose and to restore life. Re-visioning and co-creating processes of care and cure that restore all lives as one will prepare your species to restore the planet's living lungs, its water circulation, its living shade, and its evolved resilience to unexpected planetary catastrophes. By viewing life in time though an eco-centric and eco-contextualized lens that scales from your lifetime to evolutionary time, you can begin to see your world through new eyes that reveal your place in the big picture of life on earth.

Direct learning, that is, phenomenology, is essential for restoration of a living future. This method has changed with every epoch since ancient natural historians began to attempt to create views, frames, and constructs in an attempt to grasp evolving generative systems. The present moment of peril can be taken as an impetus and inspiration to engage with an exciting process of learning and problem solving that some call the living paradigm. This paradigm, which is still incubating in fields as diverse as architecture and design, agriculture, archaeology, restoration, and theology, is ripe for grass roots syncreses across outdated fields of knowledge. When you learn to cooperate with the last hundreds of millions of years of evolution while pursuing space age ways of averting asteroid collision, you will be prepared to lead your species toward sustainability and to make room for rapid human adaptation that restores evolution. Welcome to the One Life..